T0291616

HEALTH AT THE GATEWAY

**PROBLEMS AND
INTERNATIONAL OBLIGATIONS OF
A SEAPORT CITY**

HEALTH AT THE GATEWAY

PROBLEMS AND INTERNATIONAL OBLIGATIONS OF A SEAPORT CITY

BY

E. W. HOPE, O.B.E., M.D., D.Sc.

Professor of Public Health, University of Liverpool

Formerly
*Medical Officer of Health, City and Port of Liverpool;
Examiner in Public Health in the Universities of Belfast,
Cambridge, Edinburgh, London and Manchester,
and the Royal College of Physicians of London
and Royal College of Surgeons, England;
President of the Liverpool Medical
Institution and of the Society
of Medical Officers of
Health*

CAMBRIDGE
AT THE UNIVERSITY PRESS
1931

CAMBRIDGE UNIVERSITY PRESS
Cambridge, New York, Melbourne, Madrid, Cape Town,
Singapore, São Paulo, Delhi, Mexico City

Cambridge University Press
The Edinburgh Building, Cambridge CB2 8RU, UK

Published in the United States of America by Cambridge University Press, New York

www.cambridge.org
Information on this title: www.cambridge.org/9781107655652

First published 1931
First paperback edition 2013

A catalogue record for this publication is available from the British Library

ISBN 978-1-107-65565-2 Paperback

Contents

List of Illustrations

List of Illustrations

Preface

ALONG and active participation in duties associated with the advancement of the health and welfare of the people leaves no doubt that the problems involved, and the associated controversies, so fully occupy the time of those whose business it is to deal with them, that little or no opportunity is left to study the growth and results of previous endeavour. Descriptions of destructive epidemics, of bad housing, of intemperance, all resulting in conditions socially deplorable—or of imperfectly organised emigration and ineffective quarantine, resulting in international friction—are scattered and dispersed in various records. Carried forward by the stream, the workers are too engrossed to grope for its sources, and the help of a fuller knowledge of past experiences is wanting. Why, when, and how measures were put in hand, some to be abandoned as useless, others delayed while the evil grew by their lengthened toleration, and yet others carried to fulfilment with lasting benefit, would seem worth collating, and a useful service would be rendered by some review of past experiences in a form helpful to the progress of the future. It is with this definite object that this story of earlier procedure is told, and if, owing to limitations which the scope of the subject imposes, much that is worth recording finds too brief a reference, the way is pointed to sources of fuller information.

The problems have not been small, indeed it may be questioned whether the administrative body of any city and seaport in this country has been confronted with difficulties as great as those which have been successfully encountered in Liverpool—the landing within a period of six months of 300,000 destitute and fever-stricken immigrants, for example, would severely tax the administrative capacity even of the machinery of to-day.

The dismal pre-eminence resulting partly from the long neglect to regulate developments under the changing conditions of the population, and partly to happenings altogether beyond local control, did appeal with convincing force to many of the civic rulers and stimulated the foresight and beneficence of private citizens; combined voluntary and municipal effort resulted in measures which proved to be of far more than local importance, and beneficial far beyond their place of origin. This is well illustrated by the earlier sanitary legislation promoted by the Corporation of Liverpool, embracing as it did, with its additions and revisions, all phases of sanitation, since much of it after successful rehearsal in Liverpool was subsequently incorporated in the Public Health Acts. It is interesting to note too that the first appointments of a Medical Officer of Health and of Sanitary Officers, of a City Bacteriologist and of Women Health Officers, were made in Liverpool, and that it was in Liverpool that voluntary effort not only set on foot but firmly established the great work of District Nursing and the training of nurses for employment in Workhouses; the earlier day-nurseries too—the forerunners of the welfare clinics—the Society for the Prevention of Cruelty to Children, a "police-aided" clothing association to clothe destitute children, the Child Welfare Association and the first training school for the Blind, all had their birthplace in Liverpool.

The necessity for making provision for the training of prospective Health Officers of various grades made itself felt at an early period, and the means pursued to attain this end resulted in the establishment in Liverpool by civic and voluntary effort—with the inception of which the late Lord Leverhulme and the University were associated—of the first School of Hygiene in this country designed to meet the needs of those who wished to follow this branch of the Public Service. It is true that some of the Universities had already made provision for the training of the medical officer of health, and the decision of the Government in 1888, upon the recommendation of the Royal Institute of Public Health, to require from candidates for a post as medical officer of health a special Diploma in the subject, was a further stimulus in this direction; but the Liverpool School went considerably beyond this in order that the interest taken by all social workers—clergy, councillor or private citizen—should be encouraged and in various ways rendered more effective, while the City Council wisely encouraged the professional student in these matters and reaped the advantage that when in due course he joined the ranks of the medical practitioners of the City he became a valuable ally familiar with the problems.

One of the plainest functions of such a School is to ensure that the knowledge which modern sanitary science has put into our hands should be available for the masses of the people and so lead to a co-operation between them and those who are endeavouring to establish a higher standard of health and comfort— a procedure which will lessen the controversy and loss of time resulting from the criticisms of well-intentioned but ill-informed persons.

One fact obvious to those engaged in preventive medicine may be regarded either as an admirable trait in human nature or a triumph of sympathy over common sense. It is the comparative readiness with which money is given or voted for the relief or treatment of suffering, rather than for the provision of measures which would have prevented that suffering; the well-equipped ambulance at the bottom of the cliff is preferred to the fence at the top.

All seaports, home and foreign, are linked together in the common interests of health; quarantine, ancient and modern, indicates this and at the same time gives evidence of the injury to commerce resulting from ineffective and misdirected methods to attain it. Research in tropical disease has been an invaluable handmaid of sanitary science, and much is owing to Mr Joseph Chamberlain who, when Colonial Secretary, gave great encouragement to the subject.

It is not surprising that the commercial relationships of Liverpool with West African and other tropical ports brought home to those engaged in them the great risks then inseparable from residence in those regions and notably in West Africa, and stimulated the establishment in Liverpool in 1898 of the first organised School for the study of Tropical Medicine at home and in tropical areas; an action which seems appropriate in view of the wide ramifications of Liverpool commerce, reflected in the fact that more foreign countries have their consular representatives in Liverpool than in any port in the world.

It will be understood that it is not the purpose of this volume to include within its scope an account of the great work carried on by the voluntary hospitals and charities, nor to indicate the value of achievements in the treatment of disease resulting from the labours of the army of research workers at home and abroad, nor has more than the briefest allusion been possible to the help given by the clergy, especially in the poorer parts of the City, whose work has been by no means without personal risk, since many lost their lives in times of epidemic.

However wide a chasm remains to be bridged before ideals can be fulfilled, the story of the measures which have transformed the most unwholesome of sea-ports into the foremost place in sanitary administration can but be an encouragement to those whose duty it is to fulfil those aspirations; the gulf is a formidable one, but those endeavouring to bridge it are more likely to be encouraged than deterred by an acquaintance with even greater difficulties which have been overcome.

E. W. H.

UNIVERSITY OF LIVERPOOL
January 1931

FOREWORD

BY

SIR GEORGE BUCHANAN, C.B., M.D., F.R.C.P.

IF I have ventured to accept Professor Hope's invitation to add a word to this book, my only excuse lies in the desire to lay stress on the great value of the picture which he presents of the manner in which the health services of a great municipality have developed, in conception as well as in magnitude, within a single official lifetime. The records which he gives will not merely be acceptable by awaking the interested memories of contemporaries, or by providing material for some future historian; they are of definite value to the present-day student, who needs to know how the administration and practice with which he is familiar has grown up; how recently, relatively speaking, they have come about; and what kind of obstacles had to be surmounted before they were attained. They form, in fact, valuable experience to be drawn upon in the making of progress in our own day, particularly as they have been chronicled by an author who has seen the events with which he deals at first hand, and has had a share in them, so notable as that of Professor Hope during his long tenure of office in Liverpool.

These considerations apply with special force to the protection "of the gate", in other words, the port health administration of the municipality. One realises this, not only from the point of view of Government surveillance over infectious diseases in this country, but also when one is dealing with the same questions internationally at the League of Nations Health Committee or at the International Health Office in Paris. In the United States, in France, and indeed in most important maritime countries, this work has been from the outset controlled and directed from the centre; at times it has been almost the only public health service to which a Government could refer as being entirely its own. In the United Kingdom this has never been so. Central direction is necessary, and naturally has grown with the increasing interdependence of quarantine measures upon international understandings, but the public health services have throughout been those of the port sanitary authorities themselves. It is through them that the true requirements of port and health work have been ascertained, and our system has always depended on their experience, their difficulties, and the results of the battles they have fought—sometimes for the protection of the whole kingdom against the introduction of exotic infections, and sometimes (by a seeming contrast, though in fact no contrast at all) for preserving sanity and proportion when dangers of disease were exaggerated and commerce and prosperity endangered by unreasonable and uninstructed clamour. If lately, and particularly since the conclusion of the International Sanitary Convention of 1926, now almost universally ratified or accepted by the maritime powers of the world, we seem to be approaching the universal recognition of sound and scientific principles in dealing with infectious disease brought in by shipping, or with many other health questions which affect maritime commerce, it is in no small measure due to the wisdom and good epidemiological balance—using that adjective in its best sense—which, thanks to their medical services, has been traditional in the great ports of the country.

LONDON
November 1930

Chapter I

PORT ADMINISTRATION

*Evils of an insanitary Port—The Gateway of the West—
"Quarantine" a term of varying significance—Early Quarantine
in this Country—and its Failure—Origin of Bills of Health—
Renewal of Quarantine Measures—Emigration—International
Conventions—Cholera—Plague.*

THE desire for protection against avoidable disease is
common to every individual and every community; under
the name of "quarantine" it has found expression in a
changing kaleidoscope of measures in the past, and thanks to
experience and to growing knowledge is now becoming a bond
of union between nations instead of a subject of friction and
dissension. For our own country—stimulated no doubt by our
greater maritime commercial interests—may be claimed a very
large share of the credit for bringing this about; the "silver
cord" of health is the strongest in the tie which unites the
League of Nations, and the protection of a nation's health by
international agreement is an aim which meets with general
acceptance.

Whilst the risk which ports incur must correspond with the
scope of their commercial ramifications, their problems are also
concerned with the latitude and climatic conditions of the ports,
and still more with their sanitary condition, the liability to the
spread of certain infections being vastly greater under one set of
geographical circumstances than under another. An insanitary
maritime town is not only a danger to itself, but becomes
virtually a centre for diffusion of disease. The insanitary and
degrading conditions in past years of many of the maritime
towns themselves were among the reasons which led them to
exclude infected ships by quarantine, for the fruitful soil justified
only too well the dread of epidemic outbreaks. It was that
condition which led to the introduction of the then useful, if not
altogether reliable, bills of health.

The introduction of, say, plague into a well-managed British maritime town has now no serious significance so far as the health of the community is concerned; the methods adopted rob the occurrence of danger. The same observation would apply to the ports of Japan and of the United States of America, with which Liverpool, the Gateway of the West, is in constant communication, and to some other countries, whilst attention to the fulfilment of the international agreements on these matters inspires confidence and obviates trouble.

The term "quarantine" as applied to the methods adopted by communities to protect themselves against the inroads of epidemic disease is a comprehensive one; the methods, and consequently the significance of the term, have varied widely. In by-gone times it implied the complete exclusion, for a pre-scribed period (forty days), of ships, persons and merchandise coming from infected areas, without any regard whatever to the consequences which might ensue to the interests of the excluded persons or to the excluders themselves; it contemplated no possibility of ameliorative measures, and there may even be doubt whether any ameliorative measures were possible under the then existing conditions and state of knowledge.

The terrible ravages of plague in by-gone centuries in Europe account in a great measure for the rigorous application abroad of quarantine regulations for so many years, as well as for their introduction and maintenance in this country. In the fourteenth century, Venice, then at the height of her prosperity and greatness, was one of the first to establish a system of quarantine—or forty days isolation of ships—in order to prevent the spread of diseases by sea-borne commerce, the measure being directed mainly against plague.

After the Black Death had run its course, bubonic plague was never wholly absent from Europe during the next three hundred years, but no quarantine regulations were enforced in this country until 1664, when the King in Council prescribed quarantine regulations which enacted that "vessels coming from infected ports should not be permitted to come nearer than Gravesend, or such like distance, where lazarettos were ap-pointed, into which ships might discharge cargoes to be aired for forty days". Guards were appointed to prevent any communication with the shore. "After forty days, if the surgeons reported the vessel free from contagion (all apparel, goods, etcetera, having been aired in the meantime), the ship was admitted to free pratique." But these measures failed to prevent the development of the Great Plague of London in the following year.

His Majesty also issued a manifesto to his allies, informing them that "no ship or vessel would be allowed to enter port unless they brought with them a certificate from the Port Authority from whence they came". This is probably the earliest international intimation upon a health matter and the certificate was doubtless the origin of the bills of health of our own time. When plague declined, and gradually disappeared from England and Europe, the method was kept in operation against other diseases which harassed the country—smallpox, cholera, typhus, etcetera—and the basic method of quarantine by prolonged exclusion, possibly with slight modifications, was continued. But it does not appear that the practice of quarantine in the sense described was definitely established in this country by Act of Parliament until 1710 when, under the terror excited by the reappearance of plague in Poland and the Baltic areas, quarantine enactments were made which from time to time during the next half century were strengthened by further Acts of Parliament, each one placing growing burdens upon commerce. Some of them actually required British-bound vessels to undergo quarantine at certain prescribed Mediterranean and other foreign ports—the further off apparently the better—where lazarettos were provided, or even went so far as to require cargoes to be destroyed, and on occasion vessels to be burnt, compensation, however, being amply paid. Later, when vessels were permitted to perform their quarantine in the Medway, the quarantine dues often exceeded the value of the freight.

In Liverpool, up to the early part of last century, and before the days of Port Sanitary Authorities, the duty of safeguarding Britain against the inroad of epidemic infectious disease rested wholly on the Officers of H.M. Customs, who, in their turn, acted under the instructions of the Privy Council.

All ships coming from infected or suspected localities were

compelled to repair to certain appointed places, there to be detained by the Customs Authorities for periods varying from fourteen to forty days. During this period the cargoes of vessels had to be opened and aired on the decks, or on vessels provided for the purpose, and, at the expiration of the prescribed period, the vessels were permitted to discharge their goods. Cargoes were divided into two classes—so-called "enumerated" goods, cotton, wool, silk, furs, and such like porous materials which it was assumed were likely to retain infection, and "non-enumerated" goods, such as iron, timber, casks, bottles, and the like. Vessels with cargoes of non-enumerated goods, if provided with clean bills of health and having no sickness on board, were generally granted pratique almost immediately on arrival, after the necessary formalities had been observed. The presence of infectious disease or fevers of any kind, or the death of men during the voyage, caused a detention of the vessel until released by an Order in Council, whilst in the early days of the quarantine service, vessels believed to be infected with plague were not allowed within the limits of any port in the kingdom. Should they even attempt an entry they were to be driven off or sunk by gunfire. "Enumerated" goods likewise caused delay, for until these were aired both ships and goods were detained.

Early in the eighteenth century, the quarantine station in the port of Liverpool was the Sloyne, on the Cheshire side of the River Mersey, opposite Lower Bebington. Here vessels were compelled to anchor and a guard was set on shore to watch them night and day, though the guard was sometimes ineffective, and more than once men escaped from the ships under detention. In spite of the Order in Council directing the Justices of the Peace to appoint proper watchers, the guard appears to have been kept in a slovenly manner and eventually a sloop was appointed under the charge of the Admiralty to perform the duty.

By 1721 the quarantine station had been removed to Hoyle Lake (Hoylake). Here the goods were aired on board flats or lighters, provided at first by the magistrates and later by the Customs Officers, but at the cost of the merchants whose goods were concerned; naturally the merchants rebelled, and eventually, in 1771, the duty of obtaining lighters for airing goods was transferred to the Customs, the charges for their hire being defrayed by the Crown.

Many attempts were made to reduce the enormous expense thus incurred; the Commissioners of Customs endeavoured to secure the only possible island, Hilbre, at the mouth of the Dee, for land lazarettos, but the opposition of the landowners and others was too great for such a station to be secured either there or elsewhere in the Wirral peninsula. Eventually a floating lazaretto was engaged for the service and anchored in Hoyle Lake. The cargoes, however, arriving for airing more rapidly than this vessel could receive them, once more the Revenue was put to the expense of hiring lighters to supplement the lazaretto, and even this was not the end of the difficulties. Owing no doubt to the alterations in the channels of the River Dee consequent on the experiments in improving the navigation of that river, the anchorage at Hoylake began to silt up. Possibly, too, the increasing burden of vessels accelerated the inadequacy and risk of the anchorage, for whenever a gale blew from the west or north-west, no unusual experience on this coast, either the lazaretto, the flats, the vessels under quarantine, or all of them, were driven on shore and seriously damaged.

At length the Commissioners of Customs, in desperation at the ever-increasing bills for repairs to the lazaretto and the continual stream of petitions from Liverpool merchants, in 1809 appointed Bromborough Pool, above the Sloyne, as the quarantine station. No doubt the change would have been made long before but for the fierce opposition of the inhabitants of Liverpool, who feared the terrible consequences that might ensue were plague-infected ships ever to enter the river. Lighters were frequently employed at the new station, although no less than three large men-of-war and a guard-ship were stationed as permanent lazarettos within the yellow buoys which marked the quarantine anchorage. This still remains the recognised station for medical inspection for all vessels infected with plague, yellow fever, or cholera, whilst on shore adjoining is the Infectious Diseases Hospital under the control of the Port Sanitary Authority.

Some extracts from a letter addressed to the Collector of
Customs by a sub-officer on January 20, 1785, are illuminating:

Herewith you have Ten Bills for the Quarantine Service, amounting
to £264. 12s. od. for airing the enumerated Goods imported by the
'Black Queen' from Leghorn (exclusive of the Service performed by
the established Lazarette), the expense of which is upwards of £100
p. ann., a very heavy sum indeed, and the Service performed, by no
means adequate to the expense, and I cannot consistently sign them,
as it might imply that the Service has been performed agreeably to
order; the superficial manner in which the business is executed at
Hoylake (where perhaps it is done as well as at any place in the Kingdom except Standgate Creek) is not any Security for the Safety of
this Kingdom; clear I am, that when danger is apprehended, every,
the largest as well as the smallest parcel, ought to be unpacked and
opened, and the Article separated in such a manner that it may be
exposed, and for 14 days the Air to pass freely through each Article....
Importations are expected directly from the Turkish Dominion to
this Port, and from those parts where the Plague is said to have
recently raged; ...in vain are the best regulations made for the
preservation of public Health, if they are not carried *properly* into
execution—and *properly*, according to my Ideas, *where danger might
be suspected*, I never knew it done in this Port, nor can it be properly
done without incurring an amazing expense, ...and if the necessary
business cannot be done in 14 days, further time should be taken,—
this I have frequently urged, and reported when it has not been
observed....I have always considered it the business of the Officers
to observe the Order of Council, and the Honble Board's injunctions,
but in *particular*, it certainly is more incumbent on those who are
amply rewarded; and though the active part (attended with expense)
I have taken, which I am certain has been more than all other Officers
except those that watched or toiled in the Boat, has never been
considered, (and I would not now be understood that I am beating the
bush for some consideration) it has been my principle, and it shall be
my practice to obey, ...but as long as the Honble Board make the
distinction and reward you amply for mere matters of form, I am
clear the particular Care I have taken, is not expected from me, and
though in future I shall attend to the Orders in General, I shall
omit signing Bills &c. which may imply Service performed, and
deceive the Honble Board, which you, who know of the hiring of the
Vessels &c. and are paid for the Business in particular, can do.

Ar: Onslow.

The burdens became so destructive that in 1825 an amended
Quarantine Act was passed "to repeal the law relating to the

performance of quarantine and to make other provision in lieu thereof". The advantages of the Act were doubtful; it empowered the Privy Council, for the purpose of opening and airing certain classes of goods, to quarantine for forty days all vessels which had touched at places from which the Privy Council thought infection likely to be brought. The Act extended to America and the West Indies, and prescribed places where vessels should come to an anchor for the purpose of inquiry by Commissioners of Customs. Under it, so soon as the vessel had been placed in quarantine, the Officer of Customs was required to acquaint the Commissioners of Customs, and the vessel was detained until directions were given by the Privy Council. In the case of Liverpool, as the information required by the Privy Council had to be sent by mail coach, the journey, with the condition of the roads of those days, might easily occupy a week or more, and the return information another week, causing additional injury and loss.

The year 1831, when cholera was present in Europe to a very serious extent, was the last occasion of a thoroughgoing resort to quarantine of this character. The story of the progress of cholera in England in that and the two succeeding years clearly shows that quarantine failed then as hopelessly as it had failed against plague in 1664.

This failure and the results of the Reports of the Health of Towns Commission issued in 1844–5[1] revealed the urgent necessity for the establishment of a General Board of Health with skilled medical advisers, and also the encouragement of greater local activity. In due course and after much controversy, these measures were adopted. In the Report to the City Council by Drs Parkes and Sanderson referred to,[2] there is an allusion of special significance in connection with the possibilities of port sanitation; commenting on the fact that the prevalence of typhus, cholera, smallpox, or relapsing fever in distant ports, with which Liverpool shipping is in frequent communication, is followed by the introduction of these diseases, and this in turn is always attended with epidemic outbreaks, they say, "It is not possible to alter this without surrendering the commercial

[1] See p. 37.　　　　[2] See p. 99.

supremacy of Liverpool (!)—but some precautionary measures may be taken ". No doubt under the conditions which existed, and the clumsiness of the only methods available, this view was shared by the governing body, and generally accepted. However, the further suggestion that efforts should be made to obtain regular monthly reports of the health of foreign countries as regards the prevalence of epidemic disease and to be prepared for any contingency of the kind, is a forecast of port and international hygiene which has been remarkably developed in recent years.

The work of Chadwick,[1] Simon, and many others, had led up to the passing of the Public Health Act of 1872 which authorised the establishment of Port Sanitary Authorities. The gradual evolution of the powers and duties of those Authorities followed in regard to disease on board ship, the general sanitation of vessels, the care of crews and of passengers, and also the extremely important duties associated with the supervision of the cargoes.

The fact that infectious disease was constantly prevalent in Liverpool to a larger extent than elsewhere in this country, and the frequency with which it reached epidemic proportions, had long before 1872 become the subject of serious local comment and criticism; the conviction was growing that more active measures were needed to cope with the exceptional difficulties, and the view had found expression, although it was not accepted officially, that some organisation of port administration and the provision of more suitable hospital accommodation were necessary at our seaports.

Under the Public Health Act of 1872 the Local Government Board was clothed with the powers of the General Board of

[1] To Edwin Chadwick belongs the chief credit for the initiation of legislative measures for the improvement of the conditions of the poor and the conditions of the homes of the working classes. The Report of the Poor Law Commission of 1842 was largely his work, as also were the establishment of Local Authorities and provision by the Government for inspecting the administration of the sanitary law in large towns and populous districts. This latter provision, however, led to a tendency to centralisation and to a stereotyping of detail wholly inapplicable to the varied conditions of the populations, and to obstruction rather than advancement of sanitary administration. Subsequent Acts provided for fuller recognition of these varied local needs.

Health which it superseded, and empowered to constitute a Port Sanitary Authority to make special regulations dealing with diseases *not* already common to this country (exotic), as well as to provide for the treatment of persons found on arrival to be suffering from diseases which were already common to the country (endemic). In the former category were cholera, yellow fever, and plague, and in the latter such diseases as measles, smallpox, and scarlet fever.

In 1873, prior to this action being taken by the Government, the Collector of Customs had appointed a Quarantine Medical Officer to visit all ships subject to the Quarantine Code, and to him Customs Officers were required to report the presence of infectious disease. The Local Government Board, recognising the dangerous delays consequent upon such a course, discontinued this appointment, and placed the duty and responsibility upon the Medical Officer of the Port Sanitary Authority, who was thus placed in direct co-operation with the Collector of Customs.

On June 11, 1874, the Local Government Board by Provisional Order permanently constituted the Council of Liverpool the Port Sanitary Authority under the Act, and assigned to it certain powers and obligations, amongst them being powers to inspect vessels on arrival, to provide accommodation for dangerous infectious diseases, and to appoint a quarantine station, i.e. a part of the river in which vessels could anchor for the purpose of examination or detention. In consultation with Her Majesty's Customs, a suitable part of the river for such vessels as it became necessary to detain was agreed upon, and after much discussion a convenient hospital site was purchased at New Ferry with a view to accommodating cases of cholera. Upon this site the present port hospital, which has proved of such great value to all the riparian authorities, was ultimately erected. But the Council failed then to appreciate the value of the safeguards within its power to provide; as Port Sanitary Authority it decided not to appoint any officers for the purpose of inspection of vessels, on the ground that any system of inspection in regard to cleanliness would be harassing and unnecessary, the sanitary conditions being left to the Board of Trade, and all

requirements in regard to health to the Supervisor of the
Officers of Customs.

The term "quarantine" had now become a convenient one
to retain in reference to the varying methods adopted to deal
with suspected or infected vessels, with the care of those
on board suffering from infection, or who had not passed the
incubative period of that infection, and with the disinfection of
articles of commerce and of the ship herself. In the official
records we find that in the case of contagious sickness in any
vessel not under quarantine regulations a notice of the fact
would be forwarded by the Collector of Customs to the Mayor,
and be dealt with presumably by the Destitution Authorities.
"It would be wise on the apprehension of cholera to establish
an inspection, but as no permanent staff is necessary for this
purpose it will be necessary to extemporise a staff when required." The cost of nursing was to be met by the provision of
nurses when required, "a procedure," we are told, "expensive
while it lasts, but that is of very trifling consequence as the
occasions do not often arise". It was decided that all the powers
which it was possible to delegate to other riparian authorities
should be delegated, on the condition that separate hospital
accommodation should not be erected.[1]

While the requirements to make some provision for imported
infection were too reasonable to be questioned, definite official
opposition arose to the proposal to provide hospital accommodation for citizens who might be infected by dangerous
endemic infectious or epidemic diseases. The then Medical
Officer of Liverpool expressed the view "that the provision
already made by the Destitution Authority was adequate, that
the transference of this duty to a Sanitary Authority would not
only lead to enormous cost and waste of public funds, but
result in divided action in the management of the sick, and by
interference with the abstract equality of right would lead to
contentions which would inevitably assume the worst aspects of
political, social, and religious animosities and jealousies", and
further, in his opinion, "the experience of even the severest
epidemics, such as typhus in 1865, cholera in 1866, relapsing

[1] See pp. 84 *et seq.*

fever in 1870, and smallpox in 1871, does not show any necessity for supplementing the action of the Select Vestry and Boards of Guardians by any municipal interferences in the management of the sick". He writes, "I contemplate with dismay the effect of the proposed legislation in Liverpool if it should please God to visit us with a Cholera or Typhus epidemic whilst we are in a state of administrative transition".

There can be little doubt that these astonishing views, if they did not wholly reflect the opinion of the Town Council, were accepted by it, with the consequence that no attempt was made for a dozen years to provide hospital accommodation, and even then, on the score of expense, the subject was approached with reluctance. Very little further activity was shown in Liverpool in the matter until 1883, when the City Council, stimulated by the continued prevalence of typhus at home and by plague and cholera abroad, in its capacity as a Port Sanitary Authority made further port appointments, including an officer familiar with shipping to undertake inspectorial duties in connection with ships. Further medical and inspectorial appointments were subsequently made.[1] Closer attention was now paid to the sanitary conditions of vessels, crews' quarters, and to the health of the ever-increasing number of emigrants and transmigrants about to embark, as well as to their shore quarters. The health of the crews of African steamers received attention as the subject of "coast fevers" came into greater prominence—a subject subsequently investigated very fully by the Liverpool School of Tropical Medicine, founded by Sir Alfred Jones in 1898.

The prevalence of cholera in Egypt now led to conditions being imposed by an order of the Local Government Board regarding disinfection of rags imported from Egypt, which virtually led to a temporary discontinuance of such importation, and towards the end of July cargoes of rags which had already arrived in the port were stored in a railway arch which was blocked up and not opened until December when they were taken direct to vessels sailing for foreign ports, namely by 'S.S. Virginian' to Boston, U.S.A., and by other vessels to Ghent and Rotterdam.

[1] See p. 17.

The following year (1884) rags from Spain, France and Italy were excluded in view of the appearance of cholera in those countries. The arrival of the 'S.S. St Dunstan' from Marseilles, having had two deaths from cholera on board whilst en route, led to her anchorage in the quarantine ground; those of the crew who were unwell were removed to the New Ferry Hospital, fresh supplies of water were taken on board, and in two days the vessel was released after disinfection.

The next year smallpox was prevalent in Montreal and during September, October and November smallpox was imported on ten different occasions by vessels arriving from Canadian ports. In 1887 there was the rare occurrence of the arrival of cases of yellow fever on board the 'S.S. Lanfranc' from Para, the illness developing after the vessel had left that port; three of the patients died en route.

As it was already the duty of Officers of Customs to visit every incoming ship it was a natural procedure to add to their duties the highly important one of making scheduled inquiries about the health of those on board. This procedure led to various administrative improvements. In 1890 the Local Government Board embodied in a series of new regulations all the methods which had been found to be useful, and clothed the Customs and the Port Sanitary Authority with further powers in regard to dealing with suspected vessels; infected vessels, and those coming from an infected port, were required to fly a yellow flag by day and three special lights by night on coming into the river. If from the ship's log, or report of the master, the Customs Officers had reason to suspect cholera, they were empowered to detain the vessel at the approved station and communicate forthwith with the Medical Officer at the Port Office, who was required to visit the vessel at once, the Customs Officer taking him off if the Port Sanitary Authority launch was not available. If the vessel were found to be infected she was sent to the mooring station at New Ferry, the sick or suspected persons removed to the Port Hospital, and the disinfection of contacts, their clothing and the ship herself proceeded with, much on the lines which would be adopted in the case of a dwelling-house and its occupants.

As experience grew, interchanges of ideas were taking place between foreign Governments and our own, with a view to agreed standards of procedure, in order to avoid friction and dispute in regard to the methods to control infection through commercial routes.

International conventions with these aims in view had been held at Paris in 1874, Venice in 1897 and Paris in 1912, and, continued in more recent discussions, had led to interchange of information upon prevalence of disease in any one port with the Governments of other countries with which that port might trade. The scheduling of infected ports,[1] the medical examination on arrival of vessels therefrom, isolation of the sick, supervision of contacts, and disinfection, have proved their value. Obviously seaports are at present the only channels by which exotic disease can reach this country, and the sanitation of the ports themselves is therefore a matter of first consequence.

We must not forget that in the days of the panic legislation of quarantine, the knowledge of infection which we possess to-day was wanting, the connection of body vermin with typhus, of the rat and the rat flea with plague,[2] the causation of cholera and other infections, being unknown. All of them were believed to be due to aerial diffusion or a special manifestation of Divine favour or disfavour, views which still linger in regard to many diseases avoidable by human foresight.

In 1892, cholera, following upon an exceptional epidemic in British India during 1891, invaded Europe, its course taking the lines of commercial routes through Persia and Russian Turkestan into Poland, North Germany, France, Austria-Hungary and Holland. The large number of Russian emigrants passing through Prussia was regarded as a special danger, and regulations for the traffic were laid down by the German Government, as it was felt that a total prohibition of the entry of emigrants into Prussia would result in their crossing the frontier at unguarded points and by that means the advantage of their medical supervision at the frontier stations would be lost. The large emigrant

---

[1] See p. 19.
[2] During the Great Plague, dogs and cats, the natural enemies of the rat, were regarded as sources of danger and destroyed.

traffic concentrating upon the port of Hamburg was followed by the memorable outbreak of cholera there which resulted in 8605 deaths during the three months' visitation, and was the most severe from which Hamburg ever suffered. Pollution of the water supply by infected material from transmigrants was the means of infection of the population, the outbreak being virtually confined to the districts supplied by unfiltered and sewage-polluted water from the River Elbe drawn from a point below the sewer out-falls. A great number of the inhabitants fled and thus distributed the disease to many places in the Empire.

The conditions in Europe raised grave apprehensions in Liverpool, through which large numbers of emigrants were passing. Cholera reached England on August 25, 1892; the number of cases apparently was limited to thirty-five, of which eleven proved fatal. Twenty-eight of the cases came from Hamburg direct, one from Hamburg via Antwerp, three from Antwerp, two from Rotterdam, and one from Solombala near Archangel. Fortunately, cases in Liverpool were limited to four, all being emigrants who, after landing at Hull on August 26, fell sick at Liverpool on August 28. These, and the rest of their company, were isolated at the Parkhill Hospital, three of the cases only proving fatal. One emigrant en route via London died in the train. It is an interesting fact that in no instance during 1892 did the disease extend to any persons other than those arriving from abroad.

Still following the lines of traffic westward, cholera reached the United States, the history being specially interesting in view of the reimposition of the principle of the old quarantine regulations. Seven of the vessels, six carrying emigrants, which arrived in New York between August 31 and September 16, came within the definition of "infected" or "suspected". Six came from Hamburg, one from Liverpool; on five of those from Hamburg cholera had appeared, resulting in seventy-six deaths during the voyage.

The first of these vessels, the 'Moravia', arrived at New York on August 31, 1892, having had twenty-two deaths from cholera during the voyage. Upon arrival all on board were apparently in good health. The vessel was at once placed in quarantine, and the removal of the immigrants to the New York quarantine station at Hoffmann's Island ordered. Further cases of cholera subsequently occurred amongst the passengers on board this vessel.

In view of the danger of the importation of cholera to the United States by means of immigrants from infected countries stringent quarantine regulations were imposed by a circular dated September 1, issued by authority of President Harrison. It was ordered "that no vessel from any foreign port, carrying immigrants, shall be admitted to enter at any port of the United States until said vessel shall have undergone a quarantine detention of twenty days (unless such detention is forbidden by the laws of the State, or the regulations made thereunder), and of such greater number of days as may be fixed in each case by the State Authorities".

This circular was to take immediate effect, except as regards vessels already afloat, such vessels to be made the subject of special consideration. The effect of the issue of this circular was practically to suspend further shipment of immigrants to the United States.

Between September 1 and September 16, six other vessels "infected" or "suspected to be infected" with cholera arrived at New York, all hailing from Hamburg, with the exception of the 'Wyoming' from Liverpool. Each of these vessels was placed in quarantine upon its arrival, but the accommodation at the quarantine stations was found to be insufficient for the large number of persons to be dealt with, and much hardship and discomfort had to be undergone by the passengers on some of the vessels. In order to provide adequate accommodation the State acquired Fire Island as an additional quarantine station, but the inhabitants of the island and neighbouring mainland offered an armed resistance to the landing of passengers, and it was not until the militia had been called out that this resistance could be overcome.

The total number of cases of cholera reported to have occurred amongst persons arriving at New York by the seven vessels referred to was seventy-two, and of these forty-four proved fatal (one in August and forty-three in September).

The first case of cholera on land in the United States occurred in New York city on September 6, six days after cholera had appeared in the harbour, but the announcement was delayed until September 14, by which date seven cases in all had occurred, of which six had proved fatal. This delay was stated to be due to the time required for the bacteriological examination, the presence of the comma bacillus being made the diagnostic test in all cases.

Only ten cases of cholera were recorded to have taken place in New York during 1892, and of these the last case occurred on September 29. Of the ten persons attacked nine died.

The story of cholera in the United States during 1892 is remarkable in more senses than one. The ultimate result of the circular was, of course, a suspension of the emigrant traffic, but in the meantime the quarantine of many thousands of persons, nearly all in health, was deemed necessary by the State Authorities; the arrangements with a view to carrying it out were of the most rudimentary character. They had to be largely improvised on the spot, and they led to much suffering, whilst the adoption of such measures aroused a spirit of rioting, with resort to arms on the part of the neighbouring population, which had to be quelled by military measures.

Owing to the action of the United States Government considerable congestion of emigrants from the infected parts of Europe took place in Liverpool; in the meantime a number of Port Sanitary Authorities—Liverpool was not one of them— under the depressing influences of fear, were appealing to the Government to invest them with powers to place in quarantine all vessels arriving from infected ports, and even many British shipping companies urged the Government to replace the methods of dealing with infected or suspected vessels by imposing quarantine at all British ports.

The basic principles of defensive action in this country were then, and are now, a careful medical inspection of every vessel on arrival from an infected port, removal of the sick to hospital and of suspicious cases for isolation, efficient disinfection of the vessel, and the granting of permission only to healthy persons to land, upon giving their names and destinations, particulars of which were forwarded to the Medical Officers at the places to which they were travelling, in order that they should be kept under observation until all risk had passed.

It is obvious that the method is not designed to prevent the *arrival* of infection in the ports, but to deal with the vessel and its passengers on arrival in such a manner that the sick shall be cared for, the possibility of risk removed, and unnecessary interference with cargoes avoided.

The International Sanitary Convention at Venice during this year (1892) was the fifth international gathering which had met for the purpose of controlling the spread of cholera from Asia into Europe; at each one there was progressive recognition of the views put forward by the representatives of the British Government.

During the year Dr Barry, one of the inspectors of the Local Government Board, visited and made a report upon the port of Liverpool. The Port Hospital, which had been erected shortly after the constitution of the port, was now reconstructed, further accommodation provided, more suitable provision made for nurses, all auxiliaries, laundry, and offices extended, and means of access improved both from the river and the road; the appointment of two assistant Medical Officers and two additional Port Sanitary Officers was agreed upon, and arrangements were made for *medical* supervision of *every* ship coming from an infected port.

In 1893 with the march of events the constitution of the Port Sanitary Authority received further consideration, and a public inquiry was held under the chairmanship of a representative of the Local Government Board, and was attended by representatives of all riparian authorities. At this meeting, on the motion of the representative of Birkenhead, seconded by the representative of Bootle, it was unanimously decided that the City Council of Liverpool should continue to act as the Port Sanitary Authority, a decision confirmed by the Local Government Board, the apportionment of expenses resulting in a payment of approximately 80 per cent. of the cost by the City of Liverpool and the balance being divided amongst the other riparian authorities, viz. Toxteth Park, Garston, Birkenhead, Bootle, Wallasey, Lower Bebington and Bromborough.

H H   2

The opening of the Manchester Ship Canal in the following year, 1894, resulted in the constitution of a Customs Port of Manchester, and an arrangement was then made by which all Manchester-bound vessels would be examined at Liverpool by the Liverpool Port Sanitary Authority in the same way as Liverpool ships, the Manchester Authorities paying for work done on their behalf. The arrangement covered any case in which sickness on a Manchester-bound ship might break out after the vessel had passed through the port of Liverpool into the Manchester Canal. Some further adjustments of detail followed in 1897.

The Public Health Act of 1896 repealed finally what fragments still remained of the old Quarantine Act, and amplified the obligations upon masters of vessels and pilots in assisting to give effect to the 1890 Regulations in regard to cholera, yellow fever and plague. The Act also empowered the Medical Officer to visit and examine suspected vessels, or vessels coming from infected ports, whether visited by the Customs Officer or not.

From the narrow limits of a quarantine system the work of the Port Sanitary Authority has now developed into an efficient but far less irksome control over everything entering the port which may affect the public health. As our knowledge of the origin and mode of spread of disease advances, the responsibility of the Port Sanitary Authority increases, and the administrative procedure is simplified. Nowadays we are able to provide a greater degree of security against imported communicable diseases than at any previous time and with a minimum of delay and inconvenience to the trade of the port. The Mersey Docks and Harbour Board co-operates in every way with the Port Sanitary Authority, and the Mersey pilots, who usually come aboard the vessel off Point Lynas, acting under its direction, ascertain from the masters of inward-bound vessels whether they have had infectious disease on board, or whether they have touched at any of the ports on the list with which they are from time to time supplied. The pilots send wireless messages to the Port Sanitary Authority which are passed on to the Medical Officer on duty, day or night, who boards these vessels immediately on arrival in the river, and when he has taken such steps as are necessary to prevent the spread of any infection, gives the vessel permission to proceed to dock. The Port Sanitary Authority's launch is always on the river, so that vessels are expeditiously dealt with before they can enter the docks and no delay whatever is occasioned. It is also the practice of some shipping companies to notify the Port Sanitary Authority of the expected time of arrival of any of their ships from infected ports.

The Mersey Docks and Harbour Board,[1] and the various shipping and other companies occupying premises on the dock estate, co-operate with the staff of the Port Sanitary Authority in depriving rats of their harbourage.

The object of the Port Sanitary Authority is always to avoid what Sir John Simon described as "a mere irrational derangement of commerce" and "paper plausibilities", and to maintain a sound defence, based not upon fear but on scientific knowledge and common sense, against imported dangers to health, one calculated to assist rather than interfere with the trade and prosperity of the port.

The schedule of inquiries, which is in the hands of every pilot, and of every Customs Officer, varies with the information as to the prevalence of infectious sickness in foreign ports where disease is known to be endemic; some of these ports are almost permanently on the lists, which are amended in conformity with the ascertainable prevalence of disease in different parts of the world.

The sources of information are the Ministry of Health, Government Reports on the prevalence of disease, the press, shipping companies, a valuable periodical called the *United States Sanitary Record*, other American as well as British and other foreign publications, and the reports of masters and surgeons of vessels. The Port Sanitary Authority is concerned with all matters affecting the health of seamen on vessels in the port, and employs a staff of Sanitary Inspectors to visit vessels lying in the docks. The great shipping companies are solicitous for the health and comfort of seamen, and arrangements made by many of them during recent years leave little to be desired and much to be commended.

[1] See pp. 18, 26.

In the Port of Liverpool, with the growing recognition by the various riparian authorities that their interests are mutual and that their prosperity depends upon the same thing, a desire for co-operation is gradually overcoming the belief that local interests may be best served by rivalry amongst neighbours. A special Co-ordination Committee to promote these views was appointed in 1923, and considerations affecting public health, as might be expected, paved the way for agreement. So far as the medical advisers of the various Corporations on the estuary of the Mersey are concerned, perfect unanimity exists in regard to the action to be taken in connection with imported disease and the use of existing hospitals with a view to avoiding their unnecessary multiplication, as well as on such minor, but important details, as the method of notifying the Consular body and the Foreign Office through the Ministry of Health in order that international agreements, already referred to, should be complied with.[1]

With regard to the method of disinfection, for several years hydrocyanic acid gas, a highly dangerous and non-odorous gas, has been used for the purpose of disinfecting ships. An excessively poisonous agent, extreme care is necessary in its use; it is very effective in the destruction not only of rats but of insect vermin. The cost of fumigating is wholly borne by the Port Sanitary Authority, the closest attention being paid to vessels arriving from infected ports. Rats are extremely rapid breeders and the cessation of attention to any part of the dock system would result in a rapid increase in the rat population. The routine fumigation of vessels has been adopted in numerous ports, but experience has shown that thorough fumigation of vessels, in

[1] An incidental difficulty illustrates the importance attached to this notification. The obvious duty is to inform the Ministry of Health in the first instance and they in turn, through the Foreign Office, to inform the representatives of foreign Governments. These representatives on occasion turn to their Consuls in Liverpool asking why they themselves were so remiss as not to have notified the existence of disease, and imply censure which is duly passed on to the Medical Officer of Health of the port. On the other hand, if the Consuls received the first intimation, a similar question would, *mutatis mutandis*, naturally arise from the Foreign Office. Notification involves publicity through the press and those in authority prefer to receive information through the official channels; the dilemma was met by a prompt notification to each quarter through the Medical Officer of the port.

connection with which grounds for fumigation exist, is better than any half-hearted periodic fumigation, which not only gives a false sense of security, but may result in driving rats from the holds into the crews' quarters. Rat-guards, if properly applied, have been found to be efficient protection against rats leaving or boarding vessels.

The United States Quarantine Regulations until recently required that ships entering their ports should be fumigated every six months to ensure destruction of rats and so prevent danger of plague, but the expense to the Authorities and the restraint to trade led to an inquiry with a view of determining whether this regulation was absolutely necessary. A report drawn up upon a careful investigation of the condition of one hundred ships led to a modification of this regulation, and ships found free from rats by the New York inspectors are no longer compulsorily fumigated. This is an additional incentive to ship-owners to recognise that it is to their interests to eliminate rats from their ships, as then even the short detention of vessels for fumigation may be avoided.[1]

Plague

In view of the public anxiety as well as the adverse influence upon commerce which apprehensions of plague give rise to, a further reference to that subject is necessary. The endemic centres of plague have been and still are the eastern countries, notably India, China and Persia; following the lines of human intercourse, it has from time to time travelled westward—indeed to seaports in every quarter of the globe.

Visitations of plague, although at long intervals, have made deep impressions upon Great Britain, that of the fourteenth century sweeping away half the population of the kingdom. The story of the Great Plague of 1665 is well known. The belief at the time, that the King's touch was capable of effecting a cure, was a cause of some concern to the monarch himself on the ground that the exercise of this power might not be unattended by personal risk; on the other hand, it was desired that the royal dignity might not suffer, nor his miraculous powers

[1] *Lancet*, June 18, 1927, p. 1328.

be questioned and a notice to solve the difficulty was inserted in the *Intelligencer* for April 24, 1665: "This is to give notice that His Majesty hath declared His Positive Resolution not to Heal any more after the End of this Present April until Michaelmas next; and this is published to the End that all Persons concerned may take Notice thereof and not receive a Disappointment".[1]

In 1900 and 1901,[2] India and other eastern endemic centres of plague suffered more severely from that disease than usual, but Egypt, situated on the highway between East and West, had suffered very little, although the disease had made its appearance in nine separate localities in the country. Coming nearer home, a few cases were reported at Batoum, and about two dozen cases were reported at Naples. During the year 1901 no plague is known to have occurred in any other European country excepting Great Britain, where Glasgow and Liverpool were affected, each in a trifling degree. Plague had appeared in Glasgow in 1900; and it reappeared in the same part of the city in August 1901 and in October made its appearance in a different quarter at one of the city hotels. In none of these instances was the source of infection definitely traced, but in the last group of attacks plague-infected rats were found.

The wide diffusion of plague in 1900, following the lines of sea-borne communication in various quarters of the globe, led the Liverpool City Council to retain the services of medical men familiar with the disease, and also to reserve hospital beds for possible sufferers; a circular, indicating the salient features of plague, and inviting notification of every suspicious case, was forwarded to all members of the medical profession. Several cases simulating plague were reported, and on September 29, 1901, C. M., a lad aged nineteen, living in a court in Horatio Street, was admitted to the Workhouse Hospital suffering from fever and buboes which he attributed to recent injury in the football field; he died about twenty-four hours later, the cause of death being due, as confirmed by subsequent examination, to plague.

On October 23 two children named Edward and David W., living at 134 R. Street, a clean and respectable street in a some-

[1] *The Conquest of Disease,* by David Masters, p. 156.
[2] *Local Government Board Report,* 1901–2, p. 42.

what closely populated district, were reported to be suffering from typhus fever. David died within a few hours of the report being received, and Edward and a third child were removed to hospital. The illness of the children, which proved to be plague, resulted fatally on October 26 and 27, and bacteriological examination confirmed the diagnosis.

It was ascertained on close investigation in the locality that a young woman, named Margaret K., aged twenty-nine, residing at 18 E. Street in the immediate rear of the house in which the children lived, was ill. The symptoms being indicative of plague she was removed to hospital on October 27, where she recovered. Some suspicious circumstances pointing to plague were brought to light in connection with the family; Mrs K., the mother of Margaret, had died at the same address on September 28, and Rosie K., the sister of Margaret, had died there on October 3, each after a brief illness certified to be influenza, one of them having complained of tenderness under the armpits—probably axillary buboes. Mrs L., living at 82 R. Street, a friend of the K. family, who assisted in laying out the body of Mrs K., had died suddenly on October 18.

On October 26 two children named R. and B. J., aged respectively nine and seven years, were found to be ill at E. Street. They were, with their mother, removed to hospital. One of the children, Rubina J., died after a short illness, the cause of death being plague. All of these cases were connected together, either the parents being friends or the children playmates.

Besides the actual cases of plague dealt with in hospital, either members or friends in close touch with these families were isolated for observation in wards provided for the purpose, and other persons less closely associated with the sick were kept under observation at home. There was no further extension of the disease.

The reasonably comfortable circumstances of the families attacked dissociated them from the squalor and filth usually found with vermin-borne disease. The original source of the infection of these people was never conclusively traced; there was no condition in or about their dwellings to explain it, no traces of rats were found, although careful examination was made and the floors taken up. A possible means of transference of the contagion was suggested, however, by the fact that a lodger with the K. family was the officer in charge of the Princes Dock Mortuary, to which are taken the bodies of all persons—sailors, Asiatic or others—unknown or found dead, or who have died in common lodging-houses and whose friends cannot be ascertained. It is conceivable that an undiagnosed case of plague may have been conveyed to the mortuary, the officer in this way conveying the infected fleas to the house in which he lodged. The closest investigation failed to reveal any more probable explanation than this, although it must be noted that the two daughters of Mrs K., who so far as can be discovered was the earliest victim, had recently visited Glasgow in which plague existed at the time.

In this country, for administrative purposes, plague may be regarded primarily as a disease of rats which incidentally and occasionally attacks man. One species of flea forms the intermediary between the diseased rat and man; it leaves the dead or dying plague-stricken rat in search of the fresh warm blood circulating in a healthy rat or human being, and in exchange for the necessary nutriment inoculates the new host with the virus of plague. Hence the value of the large staff of trained rat-catchers employed by the Sanitary Authority.

The apprehension of plague led to many reports of doubtful cases; its actual presence increased the number. However slight the suspicion, pending confirmation, no precautions were relaxed. The Local Government Board[1] and the Consular body, at once apprised of the outbreak under the terms of the Venice Convention, were kept fully informed of the exact position of affairs.[2] A special examination of outward-bound travellers was made, emigrant houses were closely supervised and the keepers instructed as to what they were required to do; the railway companies carried out an extensive system of disinfecting carriages which had been occupied by emigrants on their way to Liverpool.

Having regard to the gravity of the points involved, it was not unnatural that the commerce of the port should to a certain

[1] Now the Ministry of Health.   [2] See p. 13.

extent be hampered, more especially as under the terms of the Venice Convention it became necessary officially to declare Liverpool an "infected" port. Owing, however, to the great personal interest taken in the circumstances by Consuls, more especially the American and French Consuls, foreign Governments were kept fully informed of the exact position of affairs, and although in one or two countries quarantine was ordered against Liverpool ships, yet, happily, this procedure was resorted to in only a few instances, and for a very limited period.

Following the wide diffusion of plague reported in the East during 1907, notably on the Chinese coast and in Japanese and Korean ports, as well as in the principal ports of Brazil and River Plate and in Lower Egypt, in several places on the Gold Coast, and over a wide area on the West Coast of South America, plague again appeared in Liverpool in the autumn of 1908. On October 23 Ernest Illage of Widnes, mate of the coal barge 'Wesley', Trafalgar Dock, who had been ailing for a couple of days, was brought in to hospital in a vehicle by his wife. On arrival the man was found to be dead. At the inquest death was ascribed to acute blood poisoning. There were, however, indications of the presence of an axillary bubo (swelling in the armpit), and bacteriological examination carried out in Liverpool and in London subsequently proved the case to have been one of plague. Meanwhile the cabin of the barge, which was found to be swarming with fleas, was thoroughly disinfected but no rats could be found. The usual proceedings were taken to keep under observation all those who had had contact with the patient or any dealings with the barge, some of them being in Widnes.

When E. Illage fell ill, a man named W. Thompson with his wife had been taken on board the barge before the disinfection of the quarters to assist in its navigation; on the morning of November 6 Mrs Thompson, in conformity with instructions to report herself if any sickness arose, came with information that her husband had been unwell throughout the night, and that she had been unable to get medical assistance for him owing to the barge being remotely placed in the dock. Thompson and his wife were removed to hospital at New Ferry, both developed plague, the man succumbed to the disease, but the woman happily recovered. The source of the first case is extremely obscure, but the infection of the other two is evident.

Apart from the loss of individual lives, the great importance of these incidents arises, not from any effect on the general public health which may ensue, but from the great commercial injury which may be done to the port unless strict observance of the terms of the Paris Convention is exercised in ports of all nations.

After an absence of plague from Liverpool for four years a case arrived on board the 'Italian Prince'; she had clean bills of health at all ports at which she loaded cargo, namely Mersina, Beyrout, Jaffa and Malta, and no plague had been reported as existing at these ports. Although no mortality amongst rats had been observed, one caught on August 1 proved to be plague-infected, as did a second rat trapped in a warehouse on August 30.

An incident showing the mischief which may arise from a disregard of international conventions and lack of observance of the conditions and procedure of British ports, received emphasis in 1912, when trouble arose with South American ports consequent upon the importation of a case of plague into Liverpool.

Previous importations of plague had been unattended with any commercial disorganisation, the long-continued vigilance on the part of the Port Sanitary Authority, the Mersey Docks and Harbour Board, the Health Department, and shipping and other companies, in their war against rats, had resulted in reducing these vermin to a minimum, but the circumstance that out of many thousands examined bacteriologically two rats were found to be infected with plague so depressed the Health Authorities of New Orleans, Galveston, and Colon, that vigorous quarantine of the by-gone type was imposed against Liverpool ships with all the rigour fear may excite. Liverpool was included in the black list of plague centres, and detention of Liverpool steamers and sulphur fumigation of the entire ship were demanded irrespective of the loss or damage to cargo which would ensue. The Sanitary Authorities of the ports named pointed out that towns, presumably in those regions, with a quarter of the population of Liverpool had on occasion claimed to have destroyed 30,000 rats, and "they term it scandalous that a great shipping centre like Liverpool should take pride in the notification that 3000 rats were caught in the various parts of the docks of Liverpool in 12 months, and it is because of this seeming slackness on the part of the Liverpool Sanitary Authorities that Liverpool has been included in the black list of plague centres". The very success which had attended these efforts proved a ground of action against Liverpool ships on the part of those uninformed of the position of affairs.

The position was described by cablegram and letter to the Authorities of New York, and to others concerned, and the Local Government Board[1] pointed out to the Foreign Office, for communication to the Governments interested, that the occurrence of a single case of plague at a port does not constitute it an infected port under the Paris Sanitary Convention. The Foreign Office further desired Sir E. Grey to take steps to assure the United States Government that there were no grounds to apprehend the introduction of plague from Liverpool, and to point out to them that the action reported to have taken place was a breach of the Paris Convention. After some delay the restrictions were removed, but the incident is important as showing the valuable part which the Consular bodies can take, were they authorised by their respective Governments to familiarise themselves with the conditions of the ports at which they are stationed.

In Liverpool, where there are Consular representatives of a larger number of foreign Governments than in any other port in the world, such an arrangement is of the first importance, notwithstanding that some of the countries which they represent have not subscribed to the international agreements.

Later in the same year, when certain restrictive measures had again been suggested by the United States Government, a memorandum issued by the Health Department of New York, whose special representative is familiar with Liverpool, says: "Our commerce with Liverpool is great in volume and value, the steamers are huge passenger liners, and the circumstances in Liverpool do not warrant the employment of measures asked for elsewhere, as the result would be to inflict an enormous damage to the commerce of the port of New York".[2]

---

[1] Now the Ministry of Health.   [2] See also Quarantine, p. 15.

In 1919, at the suggestion of the Medical Officer, an interesting investigation was made by Professor Newstead into the different species of flea found to infest rats, the object being to ascertain the extent to which the rat population harboured the particular flea responsible for the conveyance of plague. The result of the examination, so far as it had extended, showed that the special flea *capable* of carrying plague was present in nearly one fourth of the rats taken from ships, docks and warehouses adjacent thereto. In other zones of the city, excluding the dock areas, no fleas capable of carrying plague were found on the rats examined.

Summarising the position in 1920, Dr Bruce Low in a Report to the Local Government Board[1] on the progress and diffusion of plague, remarks:

Liverpool, with its large amount of shipping with the East, and with the ports of South America, is particularly liable to importation of infected rats, but the Port Sanitary Authority has so far met the danger with success, only a few instances having occurred in past years where the infection has succeeded in effecting a landing, but only for a short time, the vigorous measures hitherto employed having been always effectual in extinguishing the danger within a short period.

Liverpool's commercial relationships with every port, including plague-infected ports in various parts of the world, continue to increase, and will no doubt do so in the future. The total extinction of plague from every endemic centre is to be wished, but improbable of achievement; arrivals, therefore, of ships from plague-infected ports occasionally bringing plague-infected persons, or plague-infected rats, may be, and indeed must be looked for in the future, but the preparedness of the port to deal with incidents of the kind is a guarantee against any risk so far as the public health is concerned, and it is reasonable to believe that through the recognised channels of authoritative information—including the rapidly developing activities of the Health Section of the League of Nations, in whose counsels the experiences of Sir George Buchanan have been so helpful— these facts will be generally recognised, and incidents such as those referred to on previous pages will never recur.

[1] Now the Ministry of Health.

Chapter II

EARLIER CONDITIONS AND GROWTH
OF THE CITY

Construction of Cellar Dwellings and Narrow Streets—Absence of Sewers—Inquiries into the Health of the People—Legislation—Alcoholism.

THE dawn of the era of prosperity for Liverpool appears to have commenced as long ago as 1700 when it was a small town of 4240 inhabitants. The streets, though narrow, were separated by unbuilt-on land, but growth took the form of building closely on these spaces, and frequently on the gardens of existing houses. As the population grew denser, the margins of the brook and pool—now the Whitechapel area—were covered with human habitations, waste refuse finding its way to the waters.

In 1788 the physicians of the town brought to the notice of the Mayor and Bailiffs the trend and consequences of this development, and framed suggestions to check the growing evil which the Corporation proposed in 1802 to include in an Improvement Bill for submission to Parliament. It was thought, however, that the Bill affected the interests of certain individuals and it was not proceeded with; proposals to erect a structure for a fever hospital, and to provide a cemetery to meet growing needs, were received more favourably and acted upon.

We are indebted, about this time, to one of the numerous occasions when the burgesses of the town were in dispute with the Mayor and Bailiffs, for a fanciful description of Liverpool by Mr Erskine (subsequently Lord High Chancellor of England), who was then counsel for the Mayor and Bailiffs. That distinguished advocate refers to:

That City which stands like another Venice upon the water, which glitters with its cheerful habitations of well-protected men, which is the busy seat of trade and the gay scene of elegant amusements

growing out of its prosperity, where there are riches over-flowing and
everything which can delight a man who wishes to see the prosperity
of a great community and a great empire.... This quondam village,
which is now fit to be a proud capital for any empire in the world, has
started up like an enchanted palace even in the memory of living
man....[1]

On appeal the burgesses obtained a verdict in their favour,
under the direction of His Majesty's Court of King's Bench, "in
opposition to the eloquence of Mr Erskine, who displayed great
talent on that occasion".[2]

We turn to a perhaps truer picture, and find emphasis laid on
the *need* for "the very ample provision made by public benevolence.... The Census of 1801 finds that 2306 of the population
were living in cellars, which is rarely seen in other towns in
England, and is injurious to health. ... For want of due circula-
tion of air, inflammatory and typhus fever, and other diseases,
carry off many each year in the lower and more crowded parts
of the town". So were the foundations laid of the disease-
factories of the future.

Already explanations were sought to account for the large
numbers of burials, without at all impugning the doctrine of
the healthfulness of the place.[3]

Increase of burials [in churches] has caused many of our churches
and chapels to resemble charnel-houses rather than temples of
religious worship.... The renown of Liverpool brings in an unusual
influx of the several industrial classes of society to settle there in
search of the means of existence, some of whom, particularly from
the neighbouring kingdom, being poorly provided, and their views
frustrated, fall victims annually to disappointment, disease, and
poverty. These serve to swell the number of deaths.

That there was, however, another class, appealed to by
considerations different in character, and with very different
results, is "shown by the well known fact that on the Exchange,
not more than fifteen, out of every hundred merchants, are found
to be natives of the town".

---

[1] *Miscellaneous Pamphlets on the Conditions of Liverpool,* 1854 (Social,
Physical and Religious), vol. 66, from the Athenæum Library.
[2] *Liverpool, Its Commerce, Statistics, and Institutions,* by Henry Smithers,
1825. Dedicated to H.M. King George IV.
[3] *Ibid.*

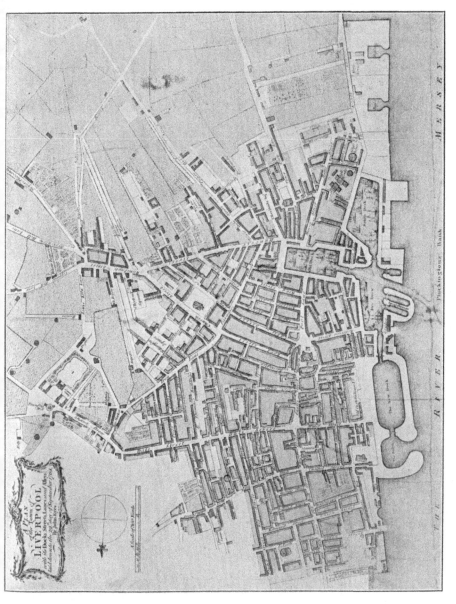

Map of Liverpool in 1768.

Their presence may have helped to explain the growing "prosperity, notwithstanding the depression caused, inter alia, by the abolition of the Slave Trade in 1807,...and...the heavy burdens of taxation, depressing the vital energies of the Nation, together with a weight of poor-rate beyond all former example, following on the long and arduous struggle with France".

Dr Currie in 1804 notes the unhealthiness of cellar dwellings, and writes that in the *new* streets a pernicious practice had been introduced of building houses to be let to labourers, in small confined courts "which have a communication with the street by a narrow aperture, but no passage for air through them, and without drainage or cleansing, and greatly overcrowded".

The Authorities, though blind to the injury to health, saw the hindrance to trade and the inconvenience to persons and vehicles passing through the narrow streets, and under Parliamentary powers expended £1500 in widening certain streets, but made no attempt to check the repetition of the same errors elsewhere. New streets followed the lines of the old crooked country lanes, and the overcrowding and packing in the heart of the town continued; back-to-back houses, arranged in narrow courts, and occupied from attic to cellar, increased rapidly, and even when, to meet the necessities of the growing population, building was carried further afield, the evils of the worst parts of the town, repeated unchecked, entailed on subsequent generations the punishment of enduring as well as the cost of rectifying them.

The chief branches of industry which found employment for skilled workers were those of porcelain and earthenware manufacture and watch-making. The domestic service difficulty in those disturbed times is not without interest to-day. It led to the formation of "A Society for the Encouragement of Servants", based upon very shrewd observations. "The complaints against servants are loud and strong. The causes thereof, I fear, frequently originate in masters and mistresses. Convince servants that you take a real interest in their welfare, and in very numerous cases duty will proceed from principle." Possibly a similar Society to-day would make an impression upon the fortress of the dole.

Nor were health matters wholly overlooked. Mr Wyke, who,

in conjunction with William Roscoe and others, was closely associated with the foundation of an institution from which sprang the Royal Institution, and ultimately the Art Gallery, also founded the first Liverpool Dispensary, the Northern, which was erected in 1829.

Dr William Moss, another contemporary writer, commenting upon the growth of the town remarks, "the annals of the history of other towns do not furnish a circumstance similar".[1] A kindly word is found for "the amazing volumes of smoke which incessantly issue from works", which "although unfavourable to vegetation, become in some respects salutary from the sulphur which it contains.... There are occasions, however, in which it is well known to be unfavourable in any degree". Even in the primitive drainage he finds a redeeming feature:

> The common sewer, it is true, is the receptacle of the dirt and filth of the town which when confined in hot weather ferments and becomes offensive. However it so happens that a quantity of *fixed air* is thrown off by this fermentation, which so far from being injurious to the human body, might if conveyed in a more agreeable manner, be desirable, and esteemed salutary.

He is sceptical as to possible harmful consequences. "If any complaints or diseases have arisen from this cause what were they, and what were the symptoms?" Yet "a stream of water occasionally (three or four times a week) in the summer season forced through it would contribute towards keeping it very sweet and clean".

Even this indulgent writer records that "the streets of Liverpool are in general narrow, and of course dirty" (why "of course"?), "both circumstances unfavourable to health.... The Corporation is an opulent one, and the health of the inhabitants deserves particular attention". The inhabitants of the poorest class live chiefly in the cellars, and insobriety results in a variety of miseries, most particularly affecting the children, who experience inattention and utter neglect.

The disposal of the dead represents the practice of the times. Reference is made to the daily custom of opening graves too early and prematurely, to make room for the remains of others.

[1] *Medical Survey of Liverpool*, William Moss, M.D.

It would appear that it was not infrequent that human remains "were, in an open public church-yard, trampled on and bandied about by a rude rabble for their pastime. The remains being dragged forth to public view and disclosed to the prying eye of wanton curiosity".

The water supply at this time was doled out to the inhabitants at the rate of one halfpenny a bucketful from carts drawn through the town. A well in Moor Street, and one known as the old Fall Well, appear to have been the chief sources of supply, although the Corporation had established waterworks as long ago as 1799.[1]

Another writer in 1823, extolling one of the public buildings, says:

The body of the building is nearly obscured by the surrounding houses which crowd upon it on all sides, and though of modern erection it has assumed a black and gloomy appearance from the smoke and filth of the neighbourhood which gives it the semblance of an ancient and neglected edifice....Several of the neighbouring streets present spectacles of vileness and misery in their lowest forms, from which the heart turns in disgust which almost overpowers the feeling of commiseration....It is deeply to be regretted that dissipation and licentiousness should almost always be the accompaniment of extensive commerce. Equally it is to be regretted that that valuable character—the British sailor—is left to indulgences which destroy the hard earned wages of the long and tedious voyage in orgies of the basest description.[2]

In 1815, Mr Rennie, the engineer, who regarded the town as better adapted for a good system of sewering than any town in the kingdom, recommended a comprehensive system. No estimation of cost was included in his recommendations, and they do not appear to have been acted upon; while public opinion was divided as to the necessity of works of this kind, administrative authority was still more divided, being shared partly by magistrates, partly by the Council, partly by Commissioners, and partly by the Poor Law Authorities, for the work was thought to be too much for any one body to discharge. The actual responsibilities of each were ill-defined, and there was no adequate public feeling to assist them. It is true that from time to time

---

[1] See p. 133.
[2] Greatorex, *Stranger in Liverpool*, 1826, Athenæum Library.

fairly comprehensive measures were put forward and discussed, but the cost was always considered an insurmountable objection, and as a consequence petty and piecemeal measures of very little value were substituted.

In 1822 paving and sewering, hitherto under the control of the Municipal Council, were vested in Commissioners. It seems that the main features of Mr Rennie's scheme were adopted in 1829 by Mr Foster, the Town Surveyor, and in 1830, under the authority of an Act of Parliament, the work of sewering was proceeded with.

The Liverpool records for the next few years are scanty but some illuminating incidents emerge, not the least being the philanthropic work done during the cholera epidemics of 1832 and 1834 by Mrs Catherine Wilkinson.[1] During these outbreaks she not only organised her kitchen into what was virtually a wash-house, but from time to time accommodated a family in a vacant room in her house whilst their own home was being disinfected. Her action drew attention to the need, and virtually paved the way, for the public wash-houses, the first of which was opened in 1841, and when these were rebuilt in 1846 Mrs Wilkinson was presented with a silver tea service by the Queen, Queen Dowager, and the ladies of Liverpool, and she and her husband were, on the suggestion of Mr William Rathbone, appointed the first superintendents.

The work of Edwin Chadwick was making itself felt, and the new Poor Law (1834), in connection with which Chadwick served as a Commissioner, was well in operation. A barrister by profession, he devoted himself to a close investigation of the conditions under which the masses of the population of the great towns were living, and his efforts resulted in an immense benefit to the health of the country.

Locally, Mr Forwood, who was associated with Poor Law administration, commenting upon the erection of what were called "cottages", i.e. small houses in courts, "each court containing 8 to 10 of them", considered them even inferior to the cellars in the wider streets. "The inhabitants keep pigs, and the magistrates have in vain endeavoured to dislodge them.

[1] See p. 142.

At the time of the cholera visitation it was discovered that pigs were frequently kept in the top rooms."[1]

Owing to the value of the land the erection of small back-to-back houses in dark and narrow courts was going on with amazing ingenuity; the scavenging was deplorable, not only there but in the main streets, the paving of which consisted chiefly of large boulder stones, with wide interstices serving as reservoirs for filth.

The Liverpool Improvement Act of 1842 contained important clauses of great variety, amongst them powers to control slaughter-houses and the inspection of meat, and the appointment of inspectors to give effect to these objects. The carrying of any part of a slaughtered animal through the streets without sufficient covering, and ill-usage in driving cattle, were forbidden by the Act;[2] the Act also prohibited bear-baiting, dog-fighting, and pastimes of a similar nature.

On a review of all that was done up to this time, we perceive no steady endeavour to carry on sanitary operations as we understand them to-day, on sound principles as preventive measures, but rather spasmodic efforts during periods of alarm, resulting in a series of patchwork expedients; conflicting authorities and conflicting interests paralysed action, and it was only in the consolidation of all power in one governing body that wholesome measures, systematically carried out, were to be looked for.

Evidence that the condition of sanitation was owing to want of knowledge rather than to the want of good intention on the part of the Council is furnished by the exhaustive investigations, made by Sidney and Beatrice Webb, of the many records dealing with the subject, largely from volumes in the Athenæum Library. In contrast with most of the other boroughs of the eighteenth century Liverpool was administered "by a capable municipal corporation with energy, dignity, and public spirit". Its attitude towards the slave trade was governed by its firm belief that the existence of the town depended on its continuance. The Liverpool Council seems to have acquiesced

---

[1] *House of Commons Enquiry into Municipal Corporations*, 1833, p. 429.
[2] See p. 196.

more readily in the passing of the Municipal Corporation Act
of 1835, under which it ceased to be a self-elective body.[1] The
Commissioners sum up the results of their inquiry as follows:
"It must be admitted that in the main the Corporation have
evinced economy and good management in their affairs. As
magistrates (its bench of Aldermen) they are attentive to their
duties, and as a governing body their conduct seems to be
materially influenced by a desire to promote welfare". It
would appear that up to 1833 such improvements as were made
—and they were many—were carried out from revenues, Liverpool being the only city in which they were not carried out by
rates.

In Liverpool a meeting was convened by the Mayor in 1845
to form a Health of Towns' Association, the main objects being
expressed in words applicable not only in that year, but applicable
in every year, even up to to-day—"to bring the subject of sanitary
reform under the notice of every class of the community, to
diffuse sound principles as widely as possible by meetings,
lectures, and publications, and especially to give information on
all points connected with the sanitary condition of Liverpool, and
the means of improving it".

On January 1, 1847, the appointment of Dr W. H. Duncan,
the first Medical Officer of Health to be appointed in this
country, was confirmed by the Town Council. Dr Duncan was
a physician to the Dispensaries and lecturer on medical jurisprudence in the School of Medicine, and the terms and conditions
of his appointment as Medical Officer were as follows:

It shall be lawful for the said Council to appoint, subject to the
approval of one of her Majesty's principal Secretaries of State, a
legally qualified medical practitioner, of skill and experience, to inspect
and report periodically on the sanitary condition of the said borough,
to ascertain the existence of diseases, more especially epidemics increasing the rates of mortality, and to point out the existence of any
nuisances or other local causes which are likely to originate and maintain such diseases, and injuriously affect the health of the inhabitants
of the said borough, and to take cognizance of the fact of the existence
of any contagious disease, and to point out the most efficacious modes
for checking or preventing the spread of such diseases, and also to

[1] *English Local Government*, by S. and B. Webb, 1908.

point out the most efficient means for the ventilation of churches, chapels, schools, registered lodging-houses, and other public edifices within the said borough, and to perform any other duties of a like nature which may be required of him; and such person shall be called the Medical Officer of Health for the Borough of Liverpool, and it shall be lawful for the said Council to pay to such officer such salary as shall be approved of by one of her Majesty's principal Secretaries of State.[1]

Anterior to this, and as a result of an inquiry in 1840, a Select Committee appointed to inquire into the circumstances of life of the inhabitants of large towns, recommended:

That it would be of the greatest advantage to the inhabitants of great towns if an inspector was appointed to enforce the due execution of sanatory regulations. They think that such an officer should (whether appointed by the rate-payers, or the guardians of the poor whom they have chosen) have the power of proceeding by indictment to abate nuisances, an old remedy of the English law, which, though somewhat in disuse, it seems quite necessary to revive and extend, to prevent and put down injury to multitudes.[2]

The Liverpool Sanitary Act, 1846, enacted:

That it shall be lawful for the said Council [the Town Council] and they are hereby required to nominate and appoint one or more persons to superintend and enforce the due execution of all duties to be performed by the scavengers appointed under this Act, and to report to the said Council and Health Committee all breaches of the by-laws, rules and regulations of the said Council and Health Committee, and to point out the existence of any nuisance, and such person shall be called "The Inspector of Nuisances".

The Reports on the Condition of the Poor, by Mr Chadwick and Dr W. H. Duncan, prior to his appointment, had previously stirred the authorities of Liverpool and attracted a wide attention. Very shortly afterwards the Commission on the Health of Towns published the result of its labours, and the public began to see that much of the misery, the moral degradation, the death, and the crime of the land, were preventable.

Liverpool was not the only city to suffer; Manchester, Leeds, Bradford, Hull, Coventry, Glasgow, and others, as well as the numerous individual townships which, aggregated together,

---

[1] Liverpool Sanitary Act, 1846.
[2] *Report on the Health of Towns*, 1840.

constitute London, were in similar plight. The only exception would appear to be Birmingham, "where the pay is better, and employment more constant than in other towns. This city, inhabited by so many industrial mechanics, so long celebrated for their skill and ingenuity, appears to form a rather striking contrast with the state of the other large towns".[1]

Alcoholism

As in the case of so many seaport towns the imprint of excessive indulgence in alcoholic drinks has in past times been heavily stamped upon Liverpool, and is commented upon by successive Medical Officers of Health and other responsible writers. Excesses, by no means restricted to rejoicings on the return of seafaring people after protracted voyages, were the occasion of the swollen records of mortality and of hospital casualties resulting from drunken brawls and criminal assault, as well as cruelty and neglect in the case of children, and above all of the extreme poverty and misery which resulted from the squandering on drink of money needed for the necessities of life. The exemption from sanitary supervision of common lodging-houses whose keepers were licensed to sell spirits was a curious privilege the evils of which have already been referred to.

In 1871 Professor Burdon-Sanderson and Professor Parkes of the Army Medical School remark: "Drunkenness and the consequent poverty, degradation and squalor, lead to starvation and beggary. The children are in rags and filth, and the unhappy people seem to know none of the comforts and few of the decencies of life, and widespread habits of drunkenness, and consequent want of food, aid their wretched homes in destroying their health".[2]

That the habit and its consequences were obstacles to the progress of sanitation long remained apparent to those really concerned with the health of the people, but the multitude of places licensed for the sale of drink, and the constant temptation which they afforded, were a lure difficult to evade, and for many years suggestions to diminish the number were resented on

[1] *Report of the Health of Towns*, 1840.
[2] See p. 33.

various grounds, such as the injury to a lawful and profitable industry. In 1883, and for a number of years following, the conditions differed little, if at all, from those described by Parkes and Sanderson, notwithstanding the remarks of Her Majesty's Judges who attributed many of the crimes of violence to this cause. A great Archbishop of York declared that he would rather see England free than England sober, but it does not appear that any menace to the freedom of England lies at the door of those workers who preferred to persist in an obstinate sobriety. The belief was gaining ground that freedom and sobriety were not necessarily divorced, and the growing efforts, educative and other, to lessen the evil were not without their effect; men and women of the stamp of Father Nugent were at work, and there were many willing to risk the odium and resentment aroused by any endeavour to limit excesses which at the same time might limit an industry.

The annual medical report dealing with the health of Liverpool for the year 1900 states that careful general observation leads to the conclusion that intemperance is diminishing. In that year, according to the evidence laid before the coroner's juries, the deaths of 236 persons, 105 of whom were women, were caused or accelerated by excessive drinking; in addition six men and four women were fatally injured whilst under the influence of drink, four inquests held in cases in which death was the result of homicidal violence showed that the person committing the deed was drunk at the time, and in three such cases both the injured person and the person who inflicted the injury were drunk at the time; in addition "alcoholism" was given as the cause of death of fourteen men and seven women. So the position merely from the point of view of direct fatality alone was serious enough, but as time went on the crippling effects upon sanitary effort were emphasised. From the point of view of waste pure and simple some interesting evidence was afforded in 1906 in connection with operations with regard to insanitary property. In one limited insanitary area in which the main characteristic of the inhabitants was extreme poverty, it was ascertained in assessing the compensation for three of the public-houses within the area that the annual receipts amounted to approximately £5000 per annum, and there were at the time forty-eight other public-houses within a radius of 200 yards of the area. Other areas furnish a similar experience; indeed in one case it was stated on behalf of the claimant firm whose extensive ownership entitled its views to consideration, "that a public-house in such a situation is situated in the best neighbourhood for the public-house trade to be found in Liverpool, and occupies a particularly commanding position, and the public were of the right sort from the point of view of customers".[1]

During this year a poster relating to the consequences of the abuse of alcohol, and approved by the Health Committee, was authorised by the City Council to be posted on the various advertising stations in the town; controversy was re-opened as to the part which alcohol had in checking improvement, many discerning much evil in any restriction which might not only injure an industry but, it was thought, fetter the freedom of the people. The Health Committee after prolonged and careful consideration of the question expressed its views on October 18, 1906, in the following resolution:

That the Health Committee begs respectfully to express its sense of the benefits resulting from the action of the Licensing Justices in diminishing the number of public-houses in the congested parts of the City; but the Committee desires respectfully to call the attention of the Licensing Justices to the injurious effects, poverty, sickness, and bad economic conditions, and loss inflicted upon the community by the continuance of the excessive and unnecessary number of public-houses in those areas which are specially dealt with by the Health Committee and by the Housing Committee of the City Council.

Public interest was aroused in the matter and on October 22 a meeting of citizens was held at St George's Hall which expressed its views as follows:

That this Meeting of Citizens, whilst recording its hearty appreciation of the past efforts of the Liverpool Bench of Magistrates to curtail the drinking facilities of the City, is deeply impressed with the conviction that it is hopeless to expect any real or permanent improvement in the areas selected by the Corporation for their re-housing operations so long as there are maintained in those areas public-

[1] *Annual Report on the Health of Liverpool*, 1912.

houses which are a constant drain on the resources of the resident population. The Meeting, therefore, respectfully urges upon the Justices the desirability of concentrating their reduction operations for a period upon such areas, in order to effect that diminution in the drinking facilities of these localities which their lamentable social condition shows to be so much and so urgently needed.

The 1906 Report of the Society for the Prevention of Cruelty to Children contains the following significant paragraph:

It is difficult, satisfactorily, to account for the misery with which the Society comes in contact—particularly as of late this question had met with considerably divided opinion—but this Committee are unable to alter theirs, which has not been arrived at hastily but is the outcome of years of experience, that the main and besetting cause is intemperance. They are fully alive to the fact that if all drunkenness ceased, degradation would still exist—but, with increased temperance and abstinence, the majority of the crime with which this Society deals would be lacking.

Children would be without clothes and food if it were not for the action of the charitable. That it is drink alone which is so largely responsible for the misery of so many children is shown by the generally admitted circumstance that it is only when those responsible for them are under the influence of drink that the children are actually ill-used and bodily injury inflicted upon them.

As a result of following to their homes very neglected children, who were at that time so frequently to be seen in the streets, the female staff in many instances were enabled to deal effectively with this form of neglect, which is almost invariably associated with the drunkenness of the mother.

During the War the restrictions—some of which very wisely have not been removed—imposed by the Defence of the Realm Act upon the manufacture and sale of intoxicants were attended with a very marked benefit which happily has been maintained. It is also noteworthy that the deaths of infants under one year of age from suffocation, owing to overlying by the mothers, has steadily and progressively diminished from 113 in 1900 to 6 in 1929. The marked reduction coincides with the restricted sale of intoxicants.

Mortality from excessive drinking is of course a crude and gross figure by which to prove the progress of temperance, but other influences even more eloquent than figures are to be found in the comfort and prosperity of districts in which so much squalor, misery and wretchedness arrested the attention. It is of interest to note that the number of "on-licences" in Liverpool in 1871 was 2317, a number gradually reduced under restrictive legislation to 1356 in 1929; the population in 1871 was 493,346 and in 1929, 874,000 (approximately).

Legislation upon this subject has been difficult and deserves the study of those interested in it, but in 1921 an Act was passed having for its main object the reducing of hours of sale and the supply and consumption of intoxicating liquor in licensed premises and registered clubs.

Chapter III

EFFORTS TOWARDS SOCIAL IMPROVEMENT

Parliamentary powers—Report of Special Commission on State of large Towns—American Civil War—Mortality from zymotic disease—359 deaths annually from typhus regarded as normal—Hospital provision—Immigration and casual unskilled labour—Emigration—Cholera on Board Ship and in the City.

THE frequency with which it has been necessary to make application to Parliament for statutory powers to enable improvements to be carried out is noteworthy, and the large number connected with water supply have already been alluded to.[1] In 1921 all preceding Acts of Parliament were consolidated into one designated the Liverpool Consolidation Act, 1921; this, of course, had the effect of obscuring the historical sequence of the various Acts and the circumstances associated with them.

The Liverpool Sanitary Act of 1846, giving certain additional powers, came into operation on January 1, 1847.[2] The year 1846 had been one of unusually high mortality, caused by the prevalence of epidemic dysentery during the summer months, followed by fever, which, however, became less prevalent in October and November; and at the close of the year the mortality of the town was rapidly subsiding to its ordinary standard. A short time previously the attention of the authorities was called to the fact that, consequent upon the potato famine in Ireland,[3] destitute and starving immigrants, driven from their cabins by the fear of starvation, were landing in Liverpool in unusual numbers. January 1, 1847, found this pauper immigration steadily increasing, and it continued in such a rapidly progressive ratio, that by the end of June not less than 300,000 had landed in Liverpool. Of these it was very moderately estimated that from 60,000 to 80,000 had located themselves in the town, occupying every nook and corner of the already overcrowded lodging-houses, and forcing their way into the cellars (about 3000 in

---

[1] See p. 141. [2] See pp. 37, 51.
[3] Thomas Carlyle, *Finest Peasantry in the World.*

number) which had been closed under the provisions of the Health Act, 1842. In different parts of Liverpool fifty or sixty of these destitute people were found in a house containing three or four small rooms, each about 12 feet by 10; and in more than one instance upwards of forty were found sleeping in a cellar.[1]

Early in February I was requested to draw up a Report, for the information of the Secretary of State, on the Health of the Town in connection with this influx. In this Report I stated that in one densely peopled district, between Scotland Road and Vauxhall Road (comprising the eastern portion of Vauxhall and Exchange Wards), in which are situated most of the lodging-houses resorted to by the immigrants, typhus fever had become more than usually prevalent; that in the other districts of the town it was not more prevalent than usual; that one-half of the whole deaths from typhus fever, since the 1st of January, had taken place in the immigrant district in question, containing about 25,000 inhabitants; that the disease affected almost exclusively the immigrants residing in crowded lodging-houses, and constituted nearly seven-eighths of all the patients in the Workhouse Fever Hospital,—five-sevenths of them from the crowded lodging-house district referred to. I added, "Should the destitute immigrants continue to flock into Liverpool as they are still doing, there can be little doubt that what we now see is only the commencement of the most severe and desolating epidemic which has visited Liverpool for the last ten years". At this time the mortality from fever was only about 18 per cent. above the average. Four months later it had risen to 2,000 per cent. above the average of former years.

In March, being again desired to report for Sir George Grey's information, I stated that there had been a progressive increase of fever in the north district mentioned in my previous report; and the epidemic had also extended to the south and central districts invaded by the immigrants, and to Scotland Ward, which were to that time comparatively free from the disease. Nearly one-half of the deaths from fever, exclusive of those in the hospital, had occurred in Exchange and Vauxhall Wards....Smallpox had appeared as an epidemic in the densely peopled immigrant districts, in the month of February; few, if any, of the children of the immigrants having been vaccinated.

It is unnecessary to trace very minutely the progress of the epidemic. Suffice it to say that hordes of sickly, half-starved, destitute people continued to pour into the town, and that fever continued to spread, *pari passu*....Had the entire population of Blackburn, Bolton, Bury, Chorley, Lancaster, Ormskirk, Prescot, Preston, Warrington, and

[1] From Report by Dr Duncan on the health of the town during the year 1847.

Wigan, taken up their residence amongst us, they would not have increased the mortality of the town more than these immigrants have done.

At this time, between 4,000 and 5,000 cases of fever, (exclusive of those in the workhouse hospital,) were under the care of the dispensary and parish medical officers,—having doubled in number since the beginning of February; the cases becoming so numerous as completely to baffle the attempts of the parish authorities to provide the requisite hospital accommodation. Hospital after hospital was opened by them in different districts of the town, the lazarettos in the river were, by consent of the Government, converted into hospital ships, and still the cases accommodated in hospital were more than twice outnumbered by those for which no hospital accommodation was provided. In the middle of April, there were 260 fever patients in hospital; in the middle of May, 800; and in the middle of June, 1,400; while nearly 4,000 in addition were under treatment at the patients' dwellings.

In the beginning of May, the epidemic burst through the barrier which had hitherto seemed to confine it to the poorer classes of the inhabitants; it invaded the better-conditioned population who had previously escaped its ravages; and gradually crept up among the wealthier classes of society. In June it appeared for the first time in Toxteth Park and West Derby. The only localities which, up to the close of the second quarter of the year, resisted the fever-poison, were Rodney Street and Abercromby Wards,—the best-conditioned districts of the town; but these, in the course of the succeeding month, succumbed to the epidemic influence.

Early in the autumn the tide of immigration had begun to slacken, and in November I reported to the committee that the inferior lodging-houses were not more crowded than usual in ordinary times.

It will be observed that the Health Authorities, as such, took little or no part in dealing with the health conditions of the times apart from the assistance generally rendered by Dr Duncan with their approval, nor had they any adequate staff for the purpose. They did, however, provide and make the fullest use of a dry-heat disinfecting station and of the public wash-houses. Dr Duncan's plea for clerical assistance, in order to enable him to give more time to actual medical duties, passed unheeded, and a correspondence, which appears to have been initiated by the Town Clerk upon instructions of the Council, in order to ascertain the number of employees in various departments, elicited the informative reply: "Dear Sir, In reply to your inquiry, I have to state that the name of the Staff of the Medical Department is William Henry Duncan".

The mortality rate from all causes during 1847[1] ranged from one out of every seven of the population in the densely populated Vauxhall district, to one in twenty-eight in the then outer areas of Rodney and Abercromby, every class of society and every locality being affected more or less. The excessive overcrowding in the worst-conditioned districts by a host of half-starved people produced results which were inevitable. In one street, Lace Street—"one of the most unhealthy streets in Liverpool, most of the cellars containing stagnant water, and all the middens undrained—not less than one third of the ordinary population of the street died in the course of the year". Losses among those working in the infected areas were heavy; ten medical practitioners, ten Roman Catholic clergymen, Church and other missionaries to the poor, a number of relieving officers, and others whose duties brought them into contact with the sick, contracted the disease and lost their lives.

But it must not be supposed that the amount of distress inflicted on the inhabitants is to be measured by the numbers who fell victims to the scourge, for I estimate that nearly 60,000 individuals suffered from Fever, and nearly 40,000 from Diarrhœa and Dysentery during that year; so that about 1 in every 3½ of the ordinary population of the borough underwent one or other form of the Epidemic.

With regard to the preventive and remedial measures adopted, it must be remembered that there had been no time to carry out any of the provisions of the Sanatory Act (1846) before the outbreak occurred. Unless a strong police or military force had been employed to guard the entrance of every cellar and every lodging-house, any attempt to enforce the powers of the Act with reference to them would have been obviously vain. But such resources as were within the reach of the Health Committee were called into play at the first outbreak of the Epidemic....Notice was given that the clothing &c. of fever patients would be washed, free of charge, at the Public Wash-houses of the Corporation. An attempt was made to induce the Irish Steam-boat Companies to increase the fare of deck passengers, but unfortunately without success until too late to be of any material benefit. The resources of private and public charity were invoked, and the appeal was freely responded to; while the Parish authorities exerted themselves to the utmost to provide the really destitute with

---

[1] Further observations from Dr Duncan's report for 1847.

the necessaries of life, as well as with ample hospital accommodation and medical attendance. But all these measures were but a drop in the bucket so long as the Irish influx continued.... The only measure at all adequate to the contingency was one which unfortunately the law did not sanction, viz., an embargo on the landing of Irish immigrants. A modified system of quarantine was indeed adopted, under sanction of the Government, about the month of July; but the only practical effect was to transfer at once to the hospital ships in the River those who were found actually suffering from fever on board the steam-boats. It is to be hoped that this disastrous year may long remain without a parallel.

The following year, 1848, saw the conclusion of the epidemic of typhus although the disease was still prevalent in non-epidemic intensity. But scarlatina, another scourge of the times, increased in severity and destroyed no less than 1516 persons, a very large majority of the sufferers being below five years of age.[1]

It is extremely probable that many of the deaths in the following year attributed to dysentery were really due to cholera, because cholera had already made its appearance in Northern Europe in 1846, and it is unlikely that it had not already reached Liverpool. Be that as it may, in 1848 it had certainly appeared in Edinburgh, Glasgow and Dumfries, approaching epidemic virulence in these towns towards the later period of the year.

Liverpool at the time was as ill-prepared to cope with an importation of cholera as it had been to cope with typhus a year before, but some arresting incidents arose in December of 1848 to which the origin of the epidemic of cholera was, rightly or wrongly, attributed. In Dr Duncan's words:

On the 10th December, an Irish family arrived in Liverpool by steamer from Dumfries, where the epidemic was then at its height. On landing, one of the children was found to be suffering from cholera, having been taken ill at the moment of embarking on board the Steamer. Both parents (the father having had premonitory diarrhœa for about a week before leaving Dumfries) were attacked with cholera on the night of their arrival in Liverpool. All three cases proved fatal, but the survivors— six in number—escaped the

---

[1] In 1927, with a population increased to more than twice the size, the deaths were twelve.

disease. On the 15th, the day subsequent to the last death,—a woman residing in the same house, who had washed the bodies of the deceased and also the bedclothes, &c., was seized with cholera and died after twelve hours' illness. These cases occurred in an unregistered lodging-house in Carlton Street....

The first undoubted case of Liverpool origin occurred on the 16th, in a crowded Irish house in a Court in Back Portland Street,—the victim being a girl about 14 years of age. On the following day, her father and a younger sister were attacked, and all three died....

"On the 18th a woman (English by birth) residing in a comparatively clean and airy apartment in Fylde Street, Toxteth Park, was taken ill and died ultimately of the consecutive fever. The distance between Back Portland Street and Fylde Street is about two miles and a half.

So far as I am aware, no further case of Asiatic cholera occurred within the borough previous to the 15th January, and certainly no death was registered from that disease.[1] There was no unusual prevalence of diarrhœa, and the health of the town appeared in all respects satisfactory. On the day mentioned, a middle-aged woman in good circumstances, residing in Eldon Street (about 300 yards from Back Portland Street), died after three days illness; and on the 21st January her husband also died, after an illness of 19 hours. The next cases occurred on the 29th and 30th January.

In addition to the foregoing cases, several others had occurred, of persons who arrived from Glasgow suffering from the disease or who were attacked within an hour or two after landing.

Cases now appeared in quick succession in Lace Street, Henry Edward Street, Saltney Street, Latimer Street, Cemaes Street, Chisenhale Street, Arley Street, and other adjacent streets well known in the history of disease, while fresh arrivals of infected persons from Glasgow and Dublin were taking place.

The epidemic spread rapidly until it attained its maximum in the middle of August when it gradually declined, and by the end of December had disappeared, having caused 6394 deaths. The mortality from all causes reached the figure of 17,047, the great

---

[1] The following case, however, must be mentioned. On the 19th December, a porter from the workhouse was sent to bring away for interment the body of the man who died in Back Portland Street on the previous night. The staircase being too narrow to admit of the coffin being taken up, the porter carried the body in his arms down the staircase to the lower room. Six or seven days afterwards this man was attacked with vomiting and purging in the workhouse and died after a short illness. The medical practitioner in attendance considered it a suspicious case, but the death was registered under the head of diarrhœa.

Efforts towards Social Improvement 49

incidence of the mortality being in the same districts in which the typhus epidemic of 1847 committed its chief ravages. The maximum mortality fell upon those between thirty and sixty years of age; a considerable excess among females is noted, and this was attributed to the greater exposure of females owing to the nature of their occupations confining them more within the immediate neighbourhood of their ill-conditioned dwellings.

Although so little was then known of the nature of cholera and of the conditions of its spread, Dr Duncan states that

However unscientific the opinion may appear it is only in cases of death and handling the secretions that there is any trustworthy evidence of danger to the attendants.... Independently of these conditions—the death of the patient and the coming in contact with the secretions—I know of no instance which supports in any way the theory of contagion.

The preventive and remedial measures recommended were, briefly, measures of general hygiene, cleanliness, improved drainage, improved dwellings, scavenging, washing of courts and streets, and so forth, and provision for early treatment on the first appearance of diarrhœa, however slight. The materials for lime-washing the courts were provided by the Board of Health, the actual work being carried out by gangs of paupers provided by the Parish Authorities. Lime-washing the exterior of the courts was unpalatable to many of the owners, who objected to it on the ground that it would deteriorate the value of their property; the occupiers, however, took a different view of the case,

Expressing themselves grateful for the improved aspect of cleanliness and cheerfulness imparted to the Courts, and with regard to the great object for which the measure was proposed—the arresting the progress of disease—the apparent effect was beyond all anticipation. I say apparent effect because other measures were in operation at the same time.

On the 18th of July the General Board of Health, the predecessor of the Local Government Board, issued an Order empowering the Medical Officer of Health to remove either the sick or the healthy from rooms occupied by one or more families where cholera or other zymotic disease had appeared, and where such step seemed necessary, in the opinion of the Officer of Health, for the protection of the other inmates. The Order of the General Board also gave power under the

H H   4 same circumstances to cause the removal of dead bodies whose retention in rooms occupied by the living might be prejudicial to health.

In only one instance was this particular power availed of, although applications made for the same purpose in upwards of thirty other instances were unnecessary, as persuasion was effective.

Measures of treatment and alleviation fell entirely within the province of the Destitution Authorities, namely the Select Vestry in the Parish of Liverpool, and the West Derby Board of Guardians in the extra-parochial districts. In addition to the workhouse hospital three auxiliary hospitals were extemporised; removals were, however, too tardy to be of benefit, and 50 per cent. of their patients died. Later in the year, too late to be of any use, a House of Refuge was opened in the Toxteth district.

As usual, the Dispensaries played an important part in providing medical relief, and notably in dealing with premonitory diarrhœa.

A large proportion of the diarrhœa cases discovered by the Visitors would in all probability have passed into cholera had it not been for the early medical aid which was thus afforded.... But the system has no power to extinguish the epidemic, as it has been thought to have, a result which no human means can bring about so long as the cholera poison continues to float in the atmosphere.

These quotations serve to illustrate the then prevalent notions concerning the nature of the disease and its mode of propagation.

As in the case of typhus, difficulties arose from the overlapping of control, and from conflicting authorities and instructions. An interesting comment arises that, in some towns visited by the cholera epidemic of this date, difficulty was experienced in obtaining the services of a sufficient number of medical advisers, non-professional persons being employed in their stead. No such difficulty in obtaining sufficient medical service existed in Liverpool, nor in constituting a Medical Relief Committee, but unfortunately there was no link connecting the Medical Relief Committee, who were acting independently, with the Board of Health and its Medical Officer, and valuable time was lost before the differences of opinion which arose as to the relative duties of the two bodies could be adjusted, and co-operation once more resumed.

On the subject of house-to-house visitation for the purpose of detecting the presence or absence of sickness, Dr Duncan emphasises the uselessness of the casual employment of illiterate persons, and insists upon the advantages of the employment of medical visitors, there being no alternative at that time between that class and the illiterate casual pauper help referred to. Trained and educated health visitors and inspectors were in the distant future, and there were no means of keeping the Medical Officer accurately informed of the actual condition in the city during the constantly recurring epidemic times, nor indeed during what were considered normal times; if there had been, the means to cope with difficulties would not have been so long delayed.

The municipal Acts of Parliament which preceded the Liverpool Act of 1847 were concerned mainly with methods of government, and the 1847 Act would appear to be the first real sanitary Act passed by Parliament, that is to say the first real Act which made specific provision with a view to facilitating scavenging, cleansing, paving, water supply, limiting the occupation of cellar dwellings, the prescription of cubic space in common lodging-houses, or houses occupied by members of more than one family, the minimum width of windows, proper arrangement of ash-pits and conveniences, the provision of baths and wash-houses, and so forth.[1]

The good example and moral effects of the revival of sanitary legislation by Liverpool, as indicated in the 1847 Act, opened a new era in sanitary legislation. Other places, encouraged by the results of the Liverpool procedure, promoted legislation, and shortly afterwards the general Towns Improvement Clauses Act, embodying most of the Liverpool provisions, became universally applicable. The Public Health Act of 1848, however, partly failed on account of excessive centralisation. The Local Board became mere collectors of taxes, the London Board being virtually the managers, but its agents sometimes had an

---

[1] *Liverpool Past and Present*, by J. Newlands, 1858. *Memorandum*, by W. T. McGowan, 1858, Athenæum Library.

interest in the work. The Local Government Act of 1858 remedied the clauses which it was thought resulted in needless interference.[1]

The census taken in 1861, the first year of office of Dr Trench, who succeeded Dr Duncan as Medical Officer of Health, revealed discrepancies between the estimated and the actual population, which have a bearing of great importance upon sanitary activity. If, for example, the population is over-estimated, the rates appear to be lower than they actually are, with the result that the need for action is not apparent. If, on the other hand, the population is under-estimated, the rates appear higher than they are, with the result that the Sanitary Authority is discouraged by the impression that effort and expenditure have been made in vain. There is, moreover, the paradox that the more successful sanitary operations are, the less apparent is the need for them.

The population of the central wards was already diminishing and the then outer areas, Everton, Kirkdale, St Anne's and Scotland wards, increasing.

The years 1859 and 1860 were prosperous years in Liverpool, with an abundance of employment and comparatively moderate prices of provisions and clothing; the prevalence of sickness and the mortality of those years (26 per 1000), which would be regarded with apprehension to-day, were then relatively good. The three succeeding years were less favourable, mainly owing to infection, a circumstance attributed to naturally recurrent cycles of healthy and sickly years. A more important association, however, was the distress which accompanied the loss of employment consequent upon the cotton famine during the American Civil War; indigent strangers and unskilled labourers from other towns, mainly in Lancashire, which were suffering from the same cause, flocked to Liverpool in vain search of employment, and swelled the ranks of the sickly and the destitute. "Benevolence did not altogether neglect, though it went dilatorily on its mission of charity to this crowd of wretchedness; for in 1861 and 1862 there was a tension of sympathy for the manufacturing operatives, and thousands of pounds were sent to other districts,

[1] Extracts from a paper by W. T. McGowan, Town Clerk, 1858

while want, misery, and sickness, abounded in our own streets."[1] This, combined with the physical, social, and administrative defects which existed in the borough, explains the outbreak of typhus which ensued in 1863, and to which 1165 deaths were certified to be due; many more certified under different names were probably due to the same cause, and indigence occasioned by the sickness and death of parents and heads of families must be added to the reckoning.

Dr Trench's Reports frequently give the impression that they reflect the views of the governing body, and, in the absence of other explanation, delays must often be ascribed to expediency. Whilst administrative energy was still concentrated on the struggle against typhus, it seems hardly to have been recognised that many of the measures taken against it were also militating against other forms of disease, for example, tuberculosis; but as more arresting epidemics declined, more adequate attention was given to other zymotics, e.g. smallpox, measles, whooping-cough, and scarlet fever. Dr Trench remarks that "Liverpool is never free from the presence of these zymotics". His views expressed the then influential public opinion "that laws necessary for the removal of their causation would too narrowly restrict the freedom of the subject", and again, "nor can we explain why the contagious principle grows occasionally virulent, or is conducted with greater facility by the atmosphere, nor why the susceptibility of the population increases, nor why the tendency of the organism to fall into this peculiar pathological state augments".

The year 1864 was no improvement upon its predecessor, the zymotics continued their destruction, typhus again heading the mortality list with 1774, although included in these deaths were a number which were probably due to enteric fever. The fact that enteric fever and typhus were distinct diseases, arising from wholly different causes, had already been proved, but in the Liverpool Register they were associated until 1883. In the sequence of their destructiveness came infantile cholera, 847 deaths; smallpox, 482; measles, 368; scarlet fever, 349; whooping-cough, 370. Multiplying the first two by 10, and the last three

[1] Trench, *Annual Report of the Health of Liverpool*, 1863.

by 20, a rough approximation to the actual number of cases may be found. No system of notification had been even thought of in this connection, and no registration existed, the only information available being a list furnished weekly by Mr Hagger, the Clerk to the Vestry, of houses whence fever patients had been removed to the workhouse by the officers of the Destitution Authority. There was no system of preventive administration in regard to these diseases, and no attempts had yet been made to obtain the information necessary as a basis of control; but in many directions Mr Hagger's efforts were of great value.

If no real effort had yet been possible to deal with the factories of disease, evidence is not wanting that the civic conscience was alert and disturbed by the condition of affairs. In November 1864, the Mayor, Mr Joseph Livingstone, and Council requested an Official Report on the subject of the prevalence of typhus. The speculations contained in the Report as to the nature of the contagion of typhus, if they neither helped nor satisfied the Mayor or Council, are interesting; a large share is ascribed "to those occult qualities of the air which Sydenham designated by the now familiar term 'epidemic constitution'". "Little is known", says the Registrar General, "of the immediate chemical or vital cause of epidemics; but in given circumstances, where many are immersed in an atmosphere of decaying organic matter, some zymotic disease is invariably produced. Where there is *starvation* it is most frequently typhus; *cold*, influenza; *heat*, cholera, yellow fever, or plague."[1] Limited truths, which appear to express the knowledge of that day.

Meanwhile the District Provident Society, and the Central Relief Society, fully confirmed the evidence that sickness and destitution, consequent upon the American War, were felt for a considerable period after the close of the struggle. The importation of cotton from China, however, and the circumstance that the rough condition of the American cotton brought by blockade runners required about three times the manipulation of cotton brought under ordinary conditions, relieved destitution by helping the labour market.

Overcrowding was still regarded as an unavoidable and un-

[1] *Report on the Health of Liverpool*, 1864.

controllable incident, rising or falling with conditions of employment, and with invasions by immigrants in search of work; besides the dislocation of the labour market occasioned by the effects of the American Civil War, long-continued east winds, keeping the homeward-bound fleet of vessels from the port, or the supervention of frost interfering with outdoor works, were important factors at the time.

The Times at this period was calling attention to the carelessness which prevailed generally in regard to convalescents. "From a most unpardonable neglect of proper purification, diphtheria, scarlatina, and typhus were caught by visitors to the lodging-houses of fashionable spas and bathing places lately occupied by convalescents from those diseases." Inferentially if things of this character were done among people of presumably higher social position, it would not be difficult to realise the obstacles in the way of the poor.

The two succeeding years, 1865 and 1866, were, from the point of view of the public health, more distressing than their immediate predecessors owing to severe visitations of typhus and cholera. In 1865 the number of deaths registered was 17,282, giving a city mortality rate of 36·4 per 1000, ranging from 41·5 per 1000 in Vauxhall, the district of highest mortality, to 19·9 in the least insanitary, namely, Rodney and Abercromby. One-half of the deaths registered occurred below five years of age. The zymotic diseases contributed 5526 deaths to swell the mortality list, typhus easily heading it with a loss of 2336 lives, and, as usual, exacting its toll mainly from middle life, with the consequent addition of large numbers of the survivors to the ranks of the destitute. The victims were almost wholly of the poorer classes, but among them were clergymen, doctors, nurses, district visitors, tradesmen (usually undertakers and pawnbrokers) and others in comfortable circumstances of life whose occupations brought them into contact with those affected.

The history of this extensive visitation follows much upon the familiar lines already described; the methods to cope with it were but slightly improved, the general sanitary administration having undergone little change, and the disease in fact exhausted itself after the infection of probably some 20,000 people.

As Dr Trench was led to remark:

Typhus may be now regarded as the constant and perennial endemic disease of large cities...fostered by the overcrowded conditions of towns enriched by commerce and manufacture; but removal and mitigation were and are within the reach of sanitary science, industry, cleanliness, forethought, and care....Always present it becomes epidemic only when the pressure of its causations had acquired force from the prostration of industry, the vices of the people, and the extension of want and indigence among the citizens....An annual average of 359 deaths may be regarded as an exceptional and favourable average of its endemic mortality. When once aroused to activity it spreads by contagion, generates an aerial influence, which physicians term "epidemic constitution", and continues its fatal progress during a certain period, independently of extraneous agencies or concomitants.

The association of typhus with poverty and of poverty with casual and unskilled employment led the Council in 1865 to appoint a committee to consider the difficulties of the type of unskilled and unorganised labour of the lowest class, and the amount of that labour available. The committee consisted of prominent men, amongst them being Messrs Jeffery, C. T. Bowring, Chairman of the Health Committee, Edward Lawrence, Edward Samuelson, James Whitty, Thomas Dover, and others. It appeared that the average earnings of the dock porters were 12s. a week, one large employer putting them as low as an average of 9s. a week, although the daily pay of 3s. 6d. would render them theoretically 21s. The intermittent arrival of vessels, sometimes in the north docks, and sometimes in the south, promptly reduced the labourers in one district or the other to destitution, and the continued influx of destitute immigrants brought down wages and living to the lowest level of wretchedness. It was suggested that if better made sanitary laws were obtained and insisted upon, a higher pay given, employment restricted to a few and made more constant, pauper immigration would cease; but the simultaneous application of these measures in all the districts affected was impossible, and the host of outcasts who slept in brick-kilns, in sheltered nooks of streets or alleys, or the pavement, where there was a chance adjunct of a baker's oven, had to be reckoned with; as a result of fatal accidents to sleepers on brick-kilns the police were instructed to deal with this evil, but the results of interference filled the bridewells to overcrowding, and the raids were discontinued. Many circumstances were passed in review, ameliorative measures considered and suggestions made by the committee.

For the next fifteen years typhus retained its endemicity, the average annual mortality being 482, ranging from 248 in the year of lowest mortality to 593 in 1881, the year of highest mortality.

The recrudescence of typhus continuing in 1882 and 1883 led the Council to appoint an additional Medical Officer; the writer, who accepted the post, found that the environment of the sufferers at that time in no way differed from the descriptions already given; filth, penury and intemperance accentuated the miseries of the sufferers; patients lay on rags in houses almost entirely bare of furniture, and starved-looking children with the usual accompaniments of destitution, filth and vermin.

Investigation threw new light on the behaviour of the disease, for example its period of incubation, the greater susceptibility of children, and the completely satisfactory results of disinfection of clothing by dry heat are explained by the now well-known fact that body vermin are the necessary intermediaries in transmitting the disease.

A further point was the mild nature of the disease in children, notwithstanding their greater susceptibility to it, quiet somnolence replacing the delirium and exhaustion of adults, so that recovery was usual.

The Guardians of the Poor still placed the workhouse institutions at the disposal of the Health Committee, but it was frequently necessary to apply to the magistrate for an order under the Public Health Act for the removal of the patient, as unwillingness to go to the workhouse hospital frequently manifested itself, and in the less poverty-stricken districts developed into a strong objection on the part of the friends; consequently the patients were treated at home, with the risk of spread of infection.

It was owing to this that the Council in 1883 decided to proceed with the provision of hospital accommodation for 50 cases of smallpox, for 200 cases of typhus, 150 of scarlet fever, and 150 for all other infectious diseases. The allocation and the disproportionate number of beds for typhus are noteworthy as indicating the expectations at the time.

There was no link connecting the medical practitioners with the Health Department, nor was there any system of notifying infections. The Notification of Infectious Diseases Act was on the Statute Book as an adoptive Act, but popular and medical sentiment in Liverpool was, in the absence of suitable hospitals, opposed to its adoption. Voluntary notifications, however, were frequently received from doctors, clergymen, school teachers, friends, and others, and were very helpful.

The Sanitary Staff was now largely increased and the training of all new officers had been such as to fit them for the special duty they were called upon to discharge.

A special officer was employed to visit at intervals of a day or two, over a period of three weeks, the houses where typhus patients had been discovered, to ascertain whether or not the rest of the family were well; any ailing member or contact was removed for isolation or kept under observation, and any necessary disinfection carried out. The system was also extended to the homes of friends and visitors of the patient, and in the event of any sickness, however trifling, appearing, a visit by the Medical Officer was paid. In this way cases were found and removed to hospital in the earliest stages of the disease and the risk of infection minimised.

Its diminution became in a measure a source of danger, since the first cases in an outbreak, usually among children, are obscure in symptoms and often escape recognition by the medical attendant, whose difficulties are increased by the dirty condition of the patient and his surroundings. The locations of the disease, however, were shifting as the old slums were demolished and the former occupants migrated to other areas less insanitary than those which they had left.

During 1903 reimportations and reappearances of typhus in the city showed the necessity for unremitting attention to the supervision of the homes of the poor. Under the administrative measures pursued, the disease declined during the next few years to very minor numbers, and except for sporadic cases, apparently due to importation, the city has remained wholly free for many years.

Reimportation of Cholera

The second of the two years 1865-6 was characterised by a visitation of cholera which resulted in a grave calamity to the city. After an absence of some ten years cholera had made its reappearance in Western Europe in the summer and autumn of 1865, but had disappeared with the approach of winter. In the absence of any international or local interchange of information it is difficult to ascertain during what month in 1866 it reappeared, but emigration was fairly active, chiefly due to Dutch and German emigrants crossing from the continent to America via Hull and Liverpool. The lodging-houses in which the emigrants were accommodated were situated in the crowded districts of the city, and very imperfectly supervised. The S.S. 'England' left the Mersey on March 28 having on board 807 emigrant passengers, and at Queenstown she received 393 more; cholera appeared on April 3, six days after sailing from Liverpool, and on April 9, when the vessel put into Halifax for additional medical assistance, there had been 92 deaths, including six of the crew. Meanwhile, on board the 'Virginia', which had left Liverpool on April 4 with 721 persons, and had completed her complement at Queenstown, cholera appeared on the eighth day after sailing and 50 deaths had occurred before the arrival of the vessel at New York on the 22nd of the month, when the passengers were removed to a quarantine vessel 'The Falcon', on which it appeared that 555 deaths subsequently occurred.

The first two deaths occurring in Liverpool were on May 2, one being a German emigrant, and the other a child of a Dutch emigrant; the families connected with these cases were intending passengers by the 'Helvetia', and upon being refused by the doctor they were directed to the workhouse hospital, but one of the patients died en route. The keeper of the emigrant lodging-house where these cases occurred held a licence for the sale of spirituous liquors, possession of which conferred upon him a privilege, namely the exclusion of the house from supervision of any kind so far as health requirements were concerned. Forty persons were lodged in a room, which allowed about 130 cubic feet for each. This was the same house to which Dr Duncan had called attention ten years previously, in which ten deaths had occurred in ten days, and fifteen deaths in the previous fortnight. "There is reason to believe", remarks Dr Trench, "that the house is frequently overcrowded, but the Committee have no control in consequence of a spirit licence being attached to the house." The Town Council was alive to the evil. "The 22nd clause of the proposed Sanitary Act gave power to deal with cases of this description, but unfortunately it was thrown out by the House of Commons, so that the evil still existed without power to remedy it." The Justices had the power to refuse the renewal of a licence in cases of this character, but they refrained, for certain reasons, from exercising it.

The 'Helvetia' left the Mersey on May 2, with 925 emigrants, of whom 527 were foreigners from various parts of Northern and Central Europe. She was to call at Queenstown for her complement, but two deaths occurred meanwhile from cholera, the patients having been lodgers in the house alluded to above. The authorities of Cork refused to admit the vessel into the harbour and she returned to Liverpool, arriving on May 4. In the absence of any system of port sanitation, and of any existing law to authorise a modified quarantine or detention, or to control the landing of passengers infected or otherwise, difficulties arose. The workhouse was the only available place for the sick, and no special means were available for their conveyance. An appeal was made to the Privy Council to authorise the detention of the ship in the river until the Medical Officer thought it safe to release her, and an order was obtained, after some delay, from the Home Secretary to prevent the landing of the sick and to control the landing of those who had been in contact with them. Two vessels, the 'War Cloud' and the 'Jessie Munn', were hired, the latter as a hospital ship, the former as a temporary place of reception for the healthy, the hospital ship being moored alongside and lashed to the 'Helvetia' for the convenience of easy removal of the sick.

Efforts were made at the same time to obtain isolated warehouses or sheds for the more permanent accommodation of emigrants during the enforced detention of the 'Helvetia'; division of nationalities and separation of the sexes engaged the first attention of the authorities, and

> The large roomy warehouses near Bankhall were rented, and then as the locality was found to be admirably suited for a sanatorium the whole of the passengers, with the exception of the sick, were removed, and as the arrangement permitted of separation of the sexes as well as the nationalities, the hospital ward was fixed up in connection with the *sanatorium*, but it was found more convenient to remove any persons having symptoms of cholera to the workhouse.

The methods adopted met with measures of success; deaths on the 'Jessie Munn' numbered 24, on the 'Helvetia' the surgeon of the vessel was the only victim. In the workhouse the deaths were 11. The 'Helvetia' was subjected to careful purification, and left on May 29 for New York and arrived without accident or a single death.

Another vessel, the 'Peruvian', sailed from Liverpool on May 15 with 758 passengers, all foreigners; 37 deaths occurred during the voyage to New York, and the vessel went to Lower Bay for quarantine; by June 12 the deaths had increased to 110, whilst 72 deaths occurred on board the 'Falcon', to which vessel a number of passengers had been transferred.

Arresting events such as these could not fail to bring into prominence the clumsiness and inefficiency of the methods relied upon to exclude imported infection from the city. The panic led to many futile suggestions; some advocated a rigid quarantine and complete exclusion of infected ships, leaving those on board to shift for themselves—indeed this proposal was to extend to all vessels coming from infected countries. These suggestions, dictated more by fear than by common sense, gave way to more reasonable measures, which in themselves indicated the germ of subsequent developments; briefly these provided, "that in case of any vessel arriving in the port having cholera on board, no person shall land from such vessel for the space of three clear days after her arrival without the permission of the local authority, and meanwhile all persons on board ship be examined by a physician or surgeon, and persons certified to be free from disease to be permitted to land". Actual sufferers were to be removed to a hospital, or designated place, and remain until certified to be free from disease, and the clothing and bedding of all persons who died of cholera were to be destroyed.[1]

The emigrants, then as now, from all parts of Europe passed through Liverpool in companies, travelling by prepaid contracts with emigration agents or companies. These contracts varied; some of them provided for the emigrants from the time they left their homes until they arrived in America, in others the emigrants catered for themselves, and consequently when delayed by illness, or other causes, the agents were not by the terms of the contract called upon to feed or provide for them, and so had no financial interest in facilitating their journey.

In Liverpool many deaths assigned to doubtful causes but associated with choleraic symptoms had been registered during June, but they were not definitely regarded as due to cholera. The first information of a death so caused of a Liverpool person was received from the Registrar on July 2 concerning Mrs Boyle, in No. 2 court, Bispham Street, a house situated in the chief fever district of the parish where the inhabitants were poorest and most squalid, and where many of the houses in the vicinity drained into adjacent open cesspools. It is uncertain when the death had occurred, but the suggestion by the relieving officer, who was dealing with the case, to induce the friends to consent to the burial of the corpse was not accepted, and the body was retained in the sitting apartment, "where men and women ate, drank and slept, the orgies of the 'wake', embracing the co-operation of scores of people, were maintained, amidst drunken and profane ribaldry, during the day and night". Dr Trench "visiting the house on the following morning found the houses crammed with men, women and children, while drunken women squatted thickly on the flags of the court before the open door of the crowded room where the corpse was laid, and the whole place reeking with tobacco smoke and the loathsome and disgusting emanations of drunken unwashed bacchanals". There is no evidence to show how Mrs Boyle herself contracted the disease, but John Boyle, the husband of the woman, and forty-eight

[1] See p. 57.

other persons within a short radius of the court, had before the end of July died from cholera. Between July 1 and July 13 the deaths attributed to cholera were 1762. It must be borne in mind that in addition to these deaths which were registered as due to cholera there were 1145 recorded from choleraic diarrhœa, probably a very large number of these being actually due to cholera.

The areas of incidence of cholera were practically the same as those of typhus and the social conditions of the people attacked were mainly the same. The climatic conditions recorded confirm Dr Trench's statement "that the subsidence of the pestilence with the first approach of wintry weather...points to the influence of heat" as a factor in the spread of the disease.

The immense proportion of cases came from the overcrowded courts and streets with only cesspool accommodation, and where dejections were retained in some nook of the occupied room. The exemplary efforts of the Select Vestry (Board of Guardians) in erecting roomy sheds for the reception of the sufferers were not in time to check the progress of contagion. The question of possible water infection at Rivington, or at the four wells which at that time supplied the borough, was very carefully considered, but no evidence found to incriminate them as sources.

Outbreaks of cholera have usually, and so frequently, been associated with contaminated water supplies, either from streams, deep or shallow wells, springs or rivers, that exceptional interest attaches to one in which the main factor was unquestionably direct infection from person to person, or possibly intermediate infection of food or drinks which were in general use.

"If we take the registry of our streets as a guide we find that it was in those which are the refuge of the destitute, the resorts of penury, the homes of vagrants, tramps and mendicants, and of our indigent population, that the cholera was earliest in its appearance, most prevalent in its intensity, and most fatal in its effect." Bispham, Lace, Fontenoy, Addison, Ford, Paul, Carlton, Saltney, Porter, and many other streets, long since demolished, are conspicuous in the list.

The renting of blocks of warehouses, provision of certain means of fumigation, disinfecting, and cleansing, were provided by the Health Committee, who also ordered "that no straw mattress or bed made of shavings, nor any articles which appeared to be almost valueless, or upon which the stains of cholera dejections were evident, should be disinfected", but set aside for valuation by an officer of the Vestry, and destroyed.

Many incidents are given illustrating the difficulty which attended any attempted removal of a corpse, or still more of a sick person; in one of the houses in Bispham Street, in which the death of a man named McAnaly had occurred, the house overlooked the cesspool, and before the funeral rites there was much drinking and excitement. An attempt to remove the corpse by force, in view of the consequences of a previous wake in the same court, led to opposition, "men and women, in maudlin and frantic drunkenness, clung to it, and howled, blasphemed, and wept". In another house in the same court the inmates, believing that the officers were going to seize the bed and bedding without payment, surreptitiously sold them, with evil consequences to the purchasers. In a cellar in the same court 'there was no furniture and the sick child was found lying on dirty straw". "In one of the cellars in this court a woman, who died of the disease, eked out a miserable existence by selling cakes and sweet-meats to children." The sale of old rags and clothing was as early as that period carried on in Paddy's Market, Bannastre Street, and contributed its share to the dissemination of infection.

In Stockdale Street the first victim was Mrs Fadden, who died on July 23. While she was suffering from cholera her neighbour, Mrs Rose Cowell, visited and helped to nurse her, and died on the same day after a very few hours illness. Rose was buried on the morning of the 25th, and while her mother attended the funeral the baby, whom she had left in the care of a friend, died in the cradle. The inspector of the district attracted by a commotion before the door of the house, found the room crowded with children who were brought by turns to kiss and pat the corpse. Among these little mourners two of the children died from cholera on July 30.[1]

[1] Report by Dr Trench, 1866.

There is no need to expand further the details of misery and squalor, but it must be remembered that the district nurses were able to render invaluable service in nursing those who were attacked.

Subsequent importations of cholera have been dealt with in the section relating to Quarantine. The importations in 1883 and in 1892, which had very minor effects so far as the health of the city was concerned, are alluded to on pp. 11 and 13.

Chapter IV

OTHER INFECTIONS

Smallpox—Modification in type—Vaccination—Special sites for Smallpox Hospitals—Scarlet Fever and Infections mainly incident upon children—Tuberculosis—Notification—Sanatoria—Infantile Cholera—Effects of Rainfall—Venereal Disease and proposed legislation—Influenza—Malaria—Hospital Accommodation—Disadvantages of unnecessary multiplication of hospitals.

DETAILS of the specific measures adopted against each of the different forms of infection would exceed the scope of this volume. Some of the general measures of sanitation directed against one proved equally effective against others, and indeed made easier the necessary specific action in each individual case; public co-operation gradually showed that the aims and results of procedure were appreciated; in the 'eighties, even among the least informed, the hospital accommodation which the Guardians provided was improved and more willingly availed of, the need lessened for a magistrate's order for compulsory removal from slum or cellar of a sufferer from typhus or smallpox, and the physical obstruction frequently associated with these removals from scores of half-drunken neighbours, involving the mild interposition of the police, gave place to a demand for removal. The educative effects of the house-to-house visitation made for the purposes of inquiry also proved beneficial in these instances.

Smallpox

The responsibilities of the Boards of Guardians included the appointment of Public Vaccinators and the administration of the Vaccination Acts; all other measures affecting the prevention and control of smallpox rested with the Sanitary Authorities.

The Vaccination Act of 1871 required all infants to be vaccinated within three months of birth, a period extended by the 1898 Act to six months, but any person who satisfied two Justices of the Peace that he conscientiously believed that the vaccination of the infant would be prejudicial to its health, received a certificate upon which the infant was allowed to remain unvaccinated. The 1907 Act required a statutory declaration only, to effect this result. Since legislation has minimised the legal obligation of vaccination it becomes correspondingly urgent that any doctor, sanitary officer, nurse, or other person whose duties, directly or indirectly, bring them within the sphere of influence of smallpox, should be so well vaccinated that this staff becomes a cordon between smallpox and those of the public susceptible to it.

It will be obvious that the only means by which an infection from which the country is free—whether it be cholera, plague, smallpox, rabies or anything else—can be re-introduced is through the ports, the aeroplane in this respect being at present negligible; hence it is that so much responsibility rests upon those controlling the sanitation of the port, a responsibility great in proportion to the magnitude of its shipping operations.[1] The procedure in dealing with a case of infection on board ship is very similar to its occurrence in a dwelling-house, and the same principles apply. In the case of smallpox, those on board are vaccinated and allowed to land after giving their names and the address of their destination, and the Medical Officer of Health of that district is apprised. The patient is removed to hospital and immediate contacts kept under observation, while the vessel is thoroughly disinfected. Importations *will* occur and there is always the possibility of persons in an incubative stage, and not yet showing any symptom of the disease, passing through the port into the country, and in this way giving rise to outbreaks, which will make the task of the Local Authorities, more especially Local Authorities of an unvaccinated community, an exceedingly difficult one.

It must be common knowledge that in every outbreak of disease the type varies in severity; just as there are mild cases and severe cases of scarlet fever or measles, there are mild cases and severe cases of smallpox. In recent years in this latter disease the mild cases have very largely predominated, a circumstance which has led to the very unwise suggestion that the mild cases should be given a different name and regarded as a

[1] See Quarantine.

different disease. It must be remembered that variation in type does not alter the nature of the disease.

In the pre-notification days the persistent nature of the infection and its insidious spread by infected persons or things led to difficulty in tracing its source. Far fewer facts from which inferences could be drawn were at the disposal of the investigator, hence it was that in the absence of sources of information now available a theory arose that smallpox was liable to be wafted long distances by air currents. Some valuable Reports upon the subject of infection were issued in 1882 by Sir Richard Thorne Thorne and Sir Henry Power which led to a wiser location of smallpox hospitals, in places in fact where surreptitious or other communication with the hospital, or its inmates, by friends or tradespeople, or by the transmission from the hospital of clothing or other articles, would be minimised.[1] The passing of the Infectious Diseases (Notification) Act in 1889 made possible more complete and effective inquiries into the question of aerial convection, and it was found that *proved* personal contact formed so conclusive an explanation of the presence of the disease as to make any other theory unnecessary.

Epidemics of former years had removed any doubt as to the spread of smallpox from ill-placed or ill-controlled hospitals, and in Liverpool the sites were carefully selected with a view to prevent unnecessary communications. The question of aerial convection, however, upon which opinion was divided for some time, was not settled until in or about 1900—and then largely upon the experiences of the Liverpool hospitals—when an action before the late Mr Justice Farwell in the Chancery Division of the High Court was brought against the Corporation of Nottingham, "to prevent the use of a site for a smallpox hospital, the objection raised practically being the question of aerial convection". The question occupied the attention of the Court for an entire week, the evidence of medical witnesses for and against was clearly put by eminent counsel, and the action against the Corporation of Nottingham failed; vigilant administration and control of a suitably placed hospital are always necessary and the result of laxity in these matters is disastrous.

[1] Sir George Buchanan, *Reports to the Local Government Board*, 1882.

The Council applied for powers to deal with friends and relatives of patients, who when inquiries were addressed to them, knowingly gave false information or knowingly suppressed the truth. Parliament granted these powers to Liverpool in 1902 and it does not appear that any other Corporation has ever possessed them. In several instances they have been of use in the application of preventive measures.

Hospital isolation has been a valuable auxiliary to other administrative and ameliorative measures in effecting the striking reduction in communicable disease shown on p. 70. These have led to the elimination of typhus, typhoid and cholera, and have robbed the not infrequent arrival in the port of such diseases as plague of any apprehension so far as the health of the community is concerned, although they still retain very great importance in view of international agreements, quarantine regulations, and so forth.[1]

Infections mainly of children

The extinction of one series of disease has resulted in a closer concentration on others, and the hospital accommodation designed originally to meet what were then regarded as the more formidable diseases became available in large measure for scarlet fever, measles, whooping-cough, diphtheria, all very formidable to children. Prolonged researches by experts and the medical profession generally into the nature and treatment of all forms of infection have contributed in no small measure to the lessened mortality shown in the table.[2]

The steady decline in mortality from scarlet fever is very marked and is due to the continuous diminution in the number of children attacked as well as to lessening in the severity of the disease. It must not, however, be forgotten that while the illness may not result fatally, the importance must be gauged rather by the possibility of consequent diseases of the heart, or ears, or elsewhere, which it may occasion.

Children of more tender age are the great sufferers from measles and whooping-cough, usually indeed of an age when

---

[1] See Quarantine. [2] See Table A.

TABLE A

The marked decline in the mortality rates from different forms of infection in Liverpool is shown by this table, which gives the *rate* per 100,000 of the population in each case during the last seven decades.

Disease		1856 to 1865	1866 to 1875	1876 to 1885	1886 to 1895	1896 to 1905	1906 to 1915	1916 to 1925	1929
	Average population	443,938	493,405	538,651	536,974	691,351	749,267	814,014	872,802
Scarlet fever	Total deaths	5,994	7,894	4,212	2,575	2,013	1,416	694	41
	Rate per 100,000 p.a.	135·0	159·9	78·1	47·9	29·1	19·0	8·5	4·7
Typhus fever	Total deaths	7,482	6,528	2,380	371	251	57	2	0
	Rate per 100,000 p.a.	168·5	132·2	44·1	6·9	3·6	0·8	0·2	0·0
Enteric fever	Total deaths	*	*	1,264	1,530	1,344	503	86	8
	Rate per 100,000 p.a.			21·5	28·4	19·3	6·7	1·5	0·9
Measles	Total deaths	3,215	4,257	5,178	3,995	3,290	4,380	3,006	427
	Rate per 100,000 p.a.	72·4	86·2	96·1	74·3	47·5	58·6	36·9	48·9
Whooping-cough	Total deaths	4,779	4,968	4,723	3,224	3,304	2,967	1,956	198
	Rate per 100,000 p.a.	107·6	100·6	87·6	60·0	47·7	39·7	24·0	21·5
Smallpox	Total deaths	1,673	2,374	908	88	195	3	4	0
	Rate per 100,000 p.a.	37·6	48·1	16·8	1·6	2·8	0·4	0·5	0·0
Diphtheria	Total deaths	*	2,129	2,434	1,655	1,955	1,239	1,366	139
	Rate per 100,000 p.a.		42·4	45·7	30·8	28·2	16·5	16·9	15·9
Phthisis	Total deaths	15,572	16,476	13,754	11,436	12,632	12,010	11,489	1,058
	Rate per 100,000 p.a.	350·7	333·9	255·3	212·9	182·7	160·7	141·1	121·2

* Records not available.

separation from the mother is very undesirable; hence the difficulty of hospital isolation in these cases, since domestic duties, the care of other children for example, prevent the mother accompanying the infected child to hospital.

These ailments are sometimes regarded as inevitable, but it is very much better that they should be postponed to the school age rather than occur in infancy when the powers of resistance are less and the results of the illness more formidable. It may be said, "Why postpone the inevitable?" but it must be realised from a moment's reflection that our whole business is to postpone the inevitable end of the length of days to which we aspire.

Tuberculosis

Many avoidable ills have contributed to Liverpool's high rate of mortality, but it was the epidemic outbreaks, notably of typhus, which awakened the public conscience and absorbed attention, since no one could be wholly free from the apprehension that he himself might be a sufferer. Although it was not recognised at the time, some of the measures adopted against typhus were operative in diminishing the ravages of tuberculosis. In the 'forties, and indeed for many years afterwards, tuberculosis was regarded as hereditary, neither the degree nor the process of its infectivity was understood; "It is", Dr Duncan remarks, "too often born with the individual and appearing at its appointed time in the palace as well as in the hovel", yet "the hereditary disposition may be augmented by habitually breathing the air of ill ventilated courts or cellars". Although progressive diminution was coincident with the slow advance of sanitation, the ravages of the disease were commented upon by Parkes and Sanderson about thirty years later; they were unable to assign any climatic conditions or special occupation as the cause, but found it rather—as all subsequent investigations have confirmed—in association with the foul atmosphere of the houses in which so many of the labouring classes were living, in the evils of irregular labour, and in the poverty and intemperance associated with it—"matters which will tax to the utmost the skill and the determination of the people of Liverpool".[1] At that time (1871) tuberculosis of the lungs destroyed 4·3 per 1000 of the population annually; then, as now, its victims were mainly those of an age of useful and productive occupation, who usually left a young family un-provided for, destitution and tuberculosis thus reacting on each other. During the first year of the extension of the Liverpool area (1895) approximately 75 per cent. of those who succumbed to this form of the disease were of the "bread-winning" age.

In 1882 Robert Koch had succeeded in isolating from tuber-culous material the specific organism—the tubercle bacillus—which actually gives rise to the disease. Still closer attention was focussed upon it at home and abroad, conferences and discussions, national and international, upon the multitudinous aspects of the scourge continued, and the transmissibility from animals, notably the tuberculous cow, was recognised. Robert Koch, who at the British Congress on Tuberculosis in London in 1901 dissented from this view, expressed his agreement with the views of other eminent bacteriologists at the Washington Congress seven years later. This form of infection, inflicting great sufferings upon children by affecting joints, bones, and other tissues, was brought into prominence, and nowhere re-ceived closer attention from the preventive and curative point of view than in Liverpool.

Following upon general principles of sanitation, and without any knowledge or even suspicion that the milk of the tuberculous cow was the cause of the tuberculous infection of the consumer, early efforts were made to deal with the neglected condition of the cowsheds. Powers were sought and obtained under the Liverpool Improvement Act of 1867 to license the premises in which the animals were kept or the milk sold, and to impose regulations upon the keepers designed with a view to safeguard the health of the animals themselves, and the Contagious Diseases (Animals) Act of 1878 further amplified these powers. With the view of bringing milk within easy reach of the poor, licences for its sale were given very freely and little supervision was exercised until several years later, when improved regulations

---

[1] *Report on the Sanitary Conditions of Liverpool*, 1871, p. 75. Drs Parkes and Sanderson.

and conferences with the Cowkeepers' Association led ultimately to a successful co-operation between the Health Authorities and that body.[1]

In order to obtain more definite information as to the extent and location of the disease a scheme of voluntary notification was inaugurated in Liverpool in 1901; this method of notification received the co-operation of the medical profession and the encouragement of the Local Government Board and at once proved valuable by bringing the sufferer into direct touch with the assistance he needed; he received from the City Health Department a card giving him simple instructions as to his mode of living, and help was given him to carry them out. Under this scheme an average of rather more than 2300 cases were notified annually until the year 1908, when the Local Government Board itself issued an order applying to the whole country, requiring the notification of all cases occurring amongst the destitute, that is of those in receipt of Poor Law Relief. Encouraged by the Liverpool experiences, and by the satisfactory results of the working of this order, the Board issued further orders in 1911 and 1912 placing tuberculosis in the same category, so far as notification is concerned, as other forms of infection; apprehension was expressed that these orders might, by exaggerating the likelihood of infection, prejudice the interests of the infected person, but it was found that the advantages to the patient, and those associated with him, far exceeded the apprehended drawbacks.

Specially arranged exhibitions, with suitable lectures, proved quite a useful method of appealing to the public. Indeed an exhibition held for a week in St Martin's Hall, Scotland Road, in the summer of 1910, attracted no less than 40,000 people, among them many specially interested, such as school teachers, nurses, milk dealers, and so forth; it was quite evident from the questions asked by those attending that the interest was very real. In 1910 the City Council appointed a specially trained Medical Officer to advise tuberculous patients how to minimise evils inherent in their home conditions and to avoid the risk of infecting others.

[1] See also pp. 192–3.

It had become evident that a large provision of sanatorium accommodation would be necessary and a start was made in 1907 by the provision of 25 beds, promptly increased to 80, at Fazakerley; 200 beds were provided in 1911 at the temporary hospital erected at Parkhill on land rented in 1885 from the Mersey Docks and Harbour Board, a close co-operation in their use being effected between the Health Department, the Poor Law Authorities and voluntary agencies. On the passing of the National Health Insurance Act in 1911 the Government appointed a Departmental Committee on Tuberculosis under the chairmanship of Mr Waldorf Astor, M.P., to report upon the subject generally. As an outcome of subsequent legislation, the City Council became the authority solely responsible for the care of the tuberculous, and in 1914 received from the Medical Officer of Health a complete "Scheme" of procedure designed to forecast the needs of the future. This received the sanction of the Local Government Board and the Insurance Commissioners.

The sanatorium accommodation at Fazakerley was soon afterwards increased to 200 beds, while a fuller use was made of voluntary institutions such as the Liverpool Sanatorium at Frodsham and the Leasowe Sanatorium for Children, opened in 1914 by the Earl of Derby, then containing 100 beds and extended later to 200. When other claims in 1924 rendered the closure of the Parkhill Sanatorium necessary, a modern building erected by the West Derby Union, the Highfield Infirmary, with 336 beds, was purchased by the Corporation from that body, and converted into the Broadgreen Sanatorium.[1] These large additions proved a great boon to the sufferers and to those associated with them, and provided the means of removing potential sources of infection.

The recovery of children admitted to the Leasowe Hospital has been remarkable. The same result followed treatment of selected cases at Heswall, West Kirby, and elsewhere, and the after-history of a large proportion shows that health has been completely re-established.

With the lessening of disease and the saving of life, the

[1] See p. 88.

anxieties to friends or relatives, who have attempted nursing under impossible home conditions aggravated by house shortage and unemployment, have been largely removed. So long ago as 1913 the Council obtained from Parliament special powers to remove and detain any sufferer from actively infective tuberculosis whose habits of life were dangerous to others, in this way following the principle of isolation of an ordinary case of infectious sickness. It has never been necessary to put this Act into operation, the moral effect of its existence being sufficient.

Provision was made under the National Insurance Act for visitation and treatment by their own doctors of those who remained at home, and home nursing was provided by arrangement with the Queen Victoria District Nursing Association. Three Tuberculosis Dispensaries provided in the "Scheme" were opened in 1912 and expert Medical Officers were appointed to each; in one case the procedure was identified with the valuable work carried on for so many years by the Liverpool Hospital for Consumption. In due course a very close co-operation developed between the tuberculosis experts and the general medical practitioners in the city; the frequency of consultations between them steadily increased and in the year 1929 the number of such consultations reached 5090—evidence of the value of the method.

The value of life saved or prolonged, or of health maintained during the productive age-period, is evident. The chart facing p. 74 shows the actual saving of life. The death-rate in the case of pulmonary tuberculosis is one-quarter what it was half a century ago, and the non-pulmonary form has diminished one-half.

The transfer to the Council of the functions hitherto discharged by the Boards of Guardians and the Insurance Committee, in connection with the treatment and prevention of tuberculosis, led naturally to a large increase in the expenditure by the Council, towards which an Exchequer grant was available. In 1912 the annual expenditure by the Council was £8000, in 1929 it was approximately £160,000, which comprises domiciliary and sanatorium treatment of adults and children, and the educational needs of the latter. The revenues received by the

Boards of Guardians and the Insurance Committee for these
purposes have been transferred to the Council.

Infantile Cholera

One of the factors most destructive of infant life in Liverpool
has been an annually recurrent epidemic of infantile cholera,
from which the sister city of Glasgow usually remained free, a
circumstance considered to be owing partly to a slightly lower
average temperature, larger water supply, and increased rainfall, and to the tenement system of dwellings which implied a
different, and, in this respect, advantageous method of refuse
removal.

The term infantile cholera has perhaps been loosely applied
and has included fatal ailments of a different character but with
choleraic symptoms. The disease has been the subject of many
investigations, one of the earliest having been made in Liverpool
during the 'eighties, at a time when insanitary surroundings
were favourable to its spread during hot and dry weather.[1] In
those times the disease usually made its appearance in June,
reached its maximum about August or September and declined
during November. The greater intensity, however, was in the
autumn, October showing a greater prevalence than June
although over a long series of years the months of June were
both drier and hotter; the autumnal rather than the early summer
conditions favoured the disease. The connection between municipal cleanliness and this form of disease is well shown by the
effects of heavy summer rain; an investigation in 1900 relating
to the preceding twenty years showed that six of them had wet
summers with an average annual rainfall of 13·8 inches and a low
annual average of 373 deaths from infantile cholera, but fourteen
of them were dry summers with an average annual rainfall of
only 10·9 inches and a high annual average of 573 deaths from
infantile cholera. The extreme years were 1891, with 16 inches
of rainfall and 203 deaths, and 1895, with 7 inches of rainfall
and 819 deaths. A higher average temperature was associated
with the seasons of low rainfall but the value of heavy rainfall in
street-washing was a great object lesson; the difference in rainfall

[1] See City Cleansing, p. 179.

in the two years 1891 and 1895 means that upwards of 900 million gallons of water were distributed in the cleansing form of rain to the then city area in the season of low mortality which were absent in the season of high mortality. The rainfall relates to the period June to September inclusive.

A wholly different element but one of equal or even greater importance was the method of feeding; a careful investigation carried out over a number of years was made into the way in which infants had been fed up to and at the time of the commencement of the illness. In those years facilities were afforded by the Vaccination Stations, which were very largely attended in various parts of the city; by visiting them when young mothers, mostly of the poorer class, were present with their babies it was easy to ascertain exactly what the common practice was in regard to infant feeding; it must be remembered, however, that in those days there were no health visitors, nor infant clinics, nor was the Notification of Births Act in existence; and it was not until nearly twenty years later that the City Council became the foster mother—or foster father—by providing supplies of suitable food. These were the days of the twilight of individual as distinct from environmental sanitation, and inquiries of this kind, cumbersome as they appear to-day, fell upon one individual, a circumstance which had at least the advantage of uniformity of standard.

In the definitely choleraic form of the disease the element of infectivity was suggested by the frequency with which the illness of the infant was accompanied, or immediately followed, by a similar illness of other members of the family, usually children. The most striking example of this occurred in connection with a Home for Foundlings which was founded by beneficent people in 1886, a large dwelling-house in Parliament Street being adapted for the reception of twelve infants. On July 1 there were ten inmates in the Home, all of whom were then, and had been previously, in ordinary health. On July 7 an infant two months old and suffering severely from choleraic symptoms was received into the Home. Within a day or two of the admission of this infant seven of the others, as well as two of the nurses, were affected. The illness proved fatal in the case of each one of the seven infants, and this melancholy event led to the closure of the Home, and postponed for many years any question of provision of a hospital for babies in Liverpool.

Whatever may have been the degree of infectivity in the homes of the poorer class, there is no doubt that food was the medium of infection. The part played by artificial feeding, which almost invariably implied improper feeding, was very clearly established. Two outstanding facts discovered by careful and prolonged inquiry may be quoted, viz. that out of 1000 consecutive deaths only thirty occurred amongst infants fed in the natural way on breast milk alone, and among equal numbers of breast fed and of artificially fed infants below three months of age born into similar surroundings, the mortality was twenty-two times as great among those artificially fed as among the breast fed, one difference being that in one case the food of the infant was never exposed to the air, and in the other it was not only unsuitable but had unavoidably been exposed to dust, putrefactive organisms, filth carried by flies, or taken from excessively foul and dirty feeding bottles, and so forth.[1] It will be observed that it was the association of heat, the season of decay and improper feeding, which brought about the results, the same method of feeding going on all the year.

The ameliorative measures then applied were almost wholly environmental, but the educational and advisory—in other words the personal or individual methods—were slowly developing, and in 1900 the Council embarked upon the task, extremely difficult but ultimately wholly successful, of actually providing a food suitable for infants at their varying ages when their mothers were not able to suckle them.[2] Other elements had to be considered, such as parental neglect or indifference, intemperate habits, or the difficulties arising from the absence of the mother,

---

[1] Cow's milk, or some preparation of it, is the best substitute for human milk no doubt, but it was no part of Nature's economy that infants should be reared by cows. The milk which Nature intended is conveyed direct to the stomach of the infant without any exposure to the air, and is free from extraneous putrefactive, or other germs; moreover, the temperature is appropriate and the various constituents suitably mixed, the latter varying with the growth of the infant, and containing elements suitable to the particular infant. These are niceties impossible to imitate in the laboratory.

[2] See p. 104.

perhaps through illness, perhaps while at work, the infant in the meanwhile being left in the custody of others, frequently another child.

As administrative methods gradually improved so the prevalence of the disease diminished. It appeared progressively later and later in the year, June and July remaining comparatively free; the peak appeared later and the decline became more rapid, retardation in appearance being accompanied by diminution in the extent of the epidemic, notwithstanding that the term in all probability now includes a variety of diseases the symptoms of which simulate infantile cholera.

The measures adopted in regard to this disease have contributed largely to the general reduction in infant mortality, and a disease which formerly headed the list of causes of the high infant mortality rates now occupies a relatively minor position.

Venereal Diseases

Those who have devoted attention to the preservation of the public health know that it is advantageous to bring known carriers of infectious diseases under control, and so to prevent the spread of those diseases.

The application of this principle has been followed by a reduction to vanishing point of some of the infectious diseases formerly rife in Liverpool, whilst the remainder have been diminished to less than one-half; the provision and application of the measures necessary to effect this control have not been simple; on the contrary, many and great difficulties had to be overcome in the procedure.

For reasons presently to be alluded to, venereal diseases have remained outside these beneficent measures of control, notwithstanding that these diseases are contagious, infectious, communicable, and dangerous to the public health, far beyond the sense in which for example scarlet fever and smallpox are, since they are transmissible to offspring, with equally damaging virulence; they are a prolific cause of sterility and of abortion, of congenital malformation and still-birth, lunacy and blindness.

The scheme at present in vogue in Liverpool had its foundation in the Report of the Royal Commission on Venereal Diseases, appointed in 1913, which, after three years of inquiry and deliberation, advised the provision of free treatment for sufferers who were willing to accept it, and facilities for accuracy of diagnosis in all cases; quackery was suppressed.

These recommendations were given effect to in Liverpool in 1917, and the methods of treatment gradually evolved with the assistance of the Local Government Board have reached a high state of efficiency. Facilities were provided in connection with hospitals and in other ways, under circumstances which would enable the patient to attend with other patients and without in any way calling attention to the nature of the illness. Various methods of propaganda—some wise, some foolish, aggressive and undesirable—were brought into operation; those of the aggressive nature happily died down and gave place to efforts more restrained and more carefully considered, and with unquestionably good results. Measures have no doubt been crippled by the absence of legal obligation upon the infected person to avail himself of or to continue treatment, and there is no penalty attached to the wilful and knowing infection of other persons, nor are there the restrictions applicable for example to measles or whooping-cough. Treatment may be discontinued at will whatever the degree of infectiousness or whatever the occupation of the infected person may be, yet continuity of treatment is of such great importance that co-operation of the sanitary centres of New York and Liverpool has been arranged to enable seamen crossing to and fro to attend at dispensaries in either place, a treatment-card carried by the patient supplying the necessary record.

An opportunity to submit the whole subject for Parliamentary consideration was afforded by the Liverpool Bill of 1920, which was already in preparation for submission to Parliament. The clauses proposed to deal with this matter were briefly: (*a*) to make it incumbent upon every infected person to seek treatment, and, in the case of feeble-minded persons, to make it the duty of the persons in charge to provide treatment for them, (*b*) to enable the Corporation to provide free treatment and suitable hospital accommodation where necessary, (*c*) to facilitate continuity of treatment and to penalise the knowing and wilful infection of others, for example young children.

The proposals received the unanimous approval of the Health Committee and of the Parliamentary Committee of the Council, as well as of the Liverpool Medical Institution. The women doctors, who have a wide experience of the ravages of the disease among women and children attending their clinics or voluntary organisations, were, without exception, favourable to the proposed clauses.

It was felt that the sanitary necessities of Liverpool were so great as to justify special application to Parliament to meet them; the port is visited by seamen of every flag and from every port throughout the world, and it is recognised that the courage which faces the perils and privations of maritime life is often reflected in recklessness where danger from venereal disease is concerned, and where the lure of the prostitute— a recognised reservoir of infection—offers exceptional facility for the interchange of these diseases.

Sight must not be lost of the fact that, apart from penal provisions, legislation is a valuable instrument of guidance and instruction—a moral deterrent to the ignorant and a restriction upon the evilly disposed; the immense moral value is too obvious to need comment.

A large amount of opinion of various religious denominations also recognises that if legislative measures are necessary to control the relatively minor impulse—say to dishonesty—they are not less necessary to restrain the overwhelming impulse— the first instinct—which ensures the perpetuation of the human race.

There are saintly people, however, not familiar with the public health aspects of the subject, who are of a contrary opinion and insist that departures from the moral life are justly punished by the infliction of disease upon others, innocent or guilty, and that the terrors of venereal disease are incentives to virtue. No sanitarian would desire any measures which would lessen the moral life; no suggestion ever has been made, nor probably ever will be made, to discard high moral teaching, or to impair influences of morality, but it cannot be accepted that either virtue or religion needs an ally so filthy and ignoble as venereal disease. It is noteworthy that in regard to the vice

HH

6

of intemperance the same school of thought adopts a wholly different attitude, and supports constructive measures for the *prevention* of intemperance (even to the extent of restricting the liberty of the inebriate), as well as for the relief of its consequences. Moral teaching should take the first place in every educational system, but it must be recognised that a duty to prevent the ravages of disease is the foremost of the obligations of the Sanitary Authority.

The proposed legislation unfortunately met with opposition, and the clauses, therefore, were not submitted for the consideration of the House of Commons.

It must be said that with the progress of experience, and thanks largely to the care and consideration shown in dealing with patients, there is now greater willingness on the part of the afflicted to seek and to continue treatment.

Influenza

The distinguishing characteristic of influenza is its tendency to assume epidemic proportions after intermittent appearance or complete absence, perhaps for a considerable period; no other disease spreads so rapidly, or affects such wide areas in so short a time. An epidemic is recorded in Liverpool during the winter of 1847–8 resulting in a special fatality to the aged and infirm—the better conditioned districts of the city being visited almost as severely as the worst conditioned; there is no record of any further epidemic visitation until that of 1891 which followed upon a world-wide outbreak, apparently arising in China. The disease was present in slight endemic form during many succeeding years, an annual average mortality of about eighty being attributed to it until 1918, when it again assumed serious epidemic proportions. The first indication of its prevalence was an unusual mortality from respiratory diseases—notably of pneumonia—a high mortality from this cause affecting coloured seamen in seamen's boarding-houses in the city. During March of the same year some cases of severe influenza were brought into the port on a vessel arriving from New York, and in April outbreaks of influenza in centres as far apart as Virginia and California showed how widespread the disease was in America at that time. Fresh importations into Liverpool occurred in considerable numbers, and the disease was popularly called the "Spanish influenza" or "Russian influenza" as extensions of the epidemic coincided with outbreaks in those countries. The epidemic rose to its maximum in Liverpool in the fourth week in October and almost simultaneously it reached its height in Paris and New York; in London the maximum mortality was reached early in November. The deaths directly attributable to influenza in Liverpool during 1918 were 1388, but the excessive number of deaths attributed to pneumonia and bronchitis left little doubt that many of them were consequent upon, and attributable to influenza as the primary factor; the fatality occurred mainly between the ages of twenty-five and sixty, which is in striking contrast to the usual incidence upon the extremes of life, viz. the very young and the aged. The great severity of the disease during pregnancy was a melancholy feature.

The epidemic continued into 1919, culminating in the first week in March, after which it rapidly declined, having occasioned a direct mortality of 1163 in less than three months, the toll from lung diseases remaining unusually high.

It is remarkable that the visitations of this scourge and the destructive results associated with them cause so little public apprehension and public anxiety; the mere presence in the city of a few cases of plague or cholera is usually the occasion for far more concern and a very groundless alarm, since they are well within the control of modern administrative methods. Happily the great epidemics of influenza occur at very long intervals, but it is usually present in endemic form and in infrequent numbers.

Malaria

It was the anxiety of merchants for the safety of employees engaged in the tropics, and notably on the West African coast, rather than risks of importation of malaria to the port, which stimulated interest and directed attention to tropical diseases; this led to the establishment of the Liverpool School of Tropical Medicine, which has taken a prominent part in the investigation and control of diseases peculiar to those countries. The development of the tropics during the last thirty years, which has been made possible by knowledge acquired by the many investigators engaged in the work, should serve as an additional stimulus to persevere with these investigations. It is not without interest to note that the malaria-carrying mosquito has been found in vessels arriving in the port of Liverpool from West Africa.[1]

Leprosy

From time to time some concern has arisen from the presence in the port of seamen and others—usually Chinese—affected in a varying degree with leprosy. These persons have been isolated until an opportunity presented itself to enable them to return to their native country.

Anthrax

Anthrax, which may be regarded as an industrial disease, is now comparatively rare. The important Anthrax Disinfecting Station for wool, under the supervision of Mr Duckering, provided by the Government in Liverpool has proved to be most effective.

Hospital Accommodation

During the long period of years in which Liverpool suffered from serious visitations of epidemic diseases, there was no appreciation of the real preventive uses of hospital accommodation, indeed the provision made was linked up with and limited to provision for the treatment of the destitute by three Boards of Guardians, namely for the Parish of Liverpool, the West Derby Area, and the Toxteth Area. The Select Vestry of the Parish of Liverpool, which was at that time by far the most important of those Boards, rendered valuable services to the city, being the first to make provision in this direction, and its

[1] Amongst other interesting descriptions of the conditions on the West Coast of Africa some 70 or 80 years ago is that of Captain Glover, the naval officer in command of the 'Day Spring', a schooner built in the Port of Liverpool specially for the Niger exploration. He speaks of "its pestilential climate—malaria, dysentery and fever taking their toll of lives, and of crews of vessels swept to death as though by a mower's scythe", and in alluding to the slave hunting habit and constant warfare of the races low in the scale of humanity, he writes of the Niger that "from its various sources until its entrance to the sea, oppression, bloodshed, and wrong blots this stream; may it please God that commerce as the means to a greater end may cover its waters with other burdens than slaves, and the results of war and depredation", a wish which has been very amply fulfilled.

willingness to do so was relied upon by the City Council, who accepted it as sufficient, and made no provision to meet the needs of the rest of the population; in later years the Boards of Guardians of the other two parishes met the needs of the destitute for whom they were responsible. Admission to the hospitals involved the disabilities then associated with Poor Law relief and an application *in formâ pauperis* had to be made, a procedure which the relatives of other than the destitute were not in the least inclined to follow, and which medical practitioners could not encourage, however desirable the removal of the patient from his surroundings might be from the point of view of limitation of infection.

The Public Health Act of 1866, already referred to, authorised the provision of a suitable hospital by the Sanitary Authority, and the removal to it, at the cost of that Authority, "of any person suffering from any dangerous or infectious disorder being without proper lodging or accommodation, or on board any ship or vessel". This definition applied only to the well-being of the patient himself, and did not have regard to risk to other people if he were not removed; the Act remained a dead letter, and could not then have been applied to any but the destitute.

It is possible that Dr Trench may have expressed the general sentiment of the Council in giving his views in 1871, five years later, upon a proposed amendment to the Act to facilitate hospital provision. He was satisfied that all necessary provision for Liverpool had been made by the Destitution Authority, and that the provision of hospital accommodation for those above the pauper class would be not only a waste of public funds, but might result in possible injury, "nor[1] did the experience of the severest epidemics show any necessity for supplementing the action of the Vestry and Boards of Guardians by municipal interference in the management of the sick.... I contemplate with dismay the effect of the proposed legislation in Liverpool if it should please God to visit us with a Cholera or Typhus epidemic whilst we are in a state of administrative transition".[2] There is small wonder that the question was wholly dropped by the Council.

[1] *Annual Health Report*, 1871.   [2] See pp. 44, 53.

In 1873, in the presence of a threatened epidemic of scarlet fever, Dr Trench suggested that the medical profession might co-operate in a larger use of the disinfecting station, and he remarks "there is every reason to believe that by rigid isolation, and by those other hygienic precautions, which as a rule are recommended by physicians, the progress of the disease might be arrested"; there is no suggestion as to where or how the "rigid isolation" could be carried into effect in the absence of any suitable hospital for the purpose, certainly not under the ordinary domestic circumstances of the sufferer.

The first move to meet the needs of people above the pauper class who had the misfortune to need hospital isolation was made about 1875 on the initiation of a few citizens (among them Dr Caton, Dr Davidson, Dr Gee, Sir Arthur Forwood, Mr Christopher Bushell, and Mr Paget), who rented a large private house in Netherfield Road to meet the needs of persons arriving in the port, or young people in business houses, residents in schools, and others, and the Council in 1880 granted a subsidy of £250 per annum towards the cost provided that twenty-five beds were placed at the disposal of the Medical Officer of Health at the reduced cost of 7s. per week, in this way recognising its responsibility in the matter; this action, however, did not even fringe the difficulty, and in 1883 the Council were still without one single bed for the isolation of infection, or for any other purpose, no matter what the necessities of the case, or the social position of the patient. The opposition to procedure arose from those who recognised the cost but not the necessity for incurring it; much discussion and a multitude of proposals led the Council in the following year to appeal to the Liverpool Medical Institution for guidance as to the number of beds necessary. At that time the relationships between the medical profession and the Health Department were far from happy, owing largely to an attempt to introduce the Notification of Infectious Diseases Act at a time when no machinery existed to give effect to it and no useful result could follow, and when, among other grievances, that of sufficient hospital accommodation was unremedied.

The advice given to provide 400 beds forthwith was not

accepted, but deputations were appointed by the Council to visit various towns to see what was being done elsewhere.

Evidence sufficiently strong to convince the doubters of the preventive value of hospital isolation of infected persons was provided by administrative developments in 1883 and a few succeeding years, and mainly in relation to typhus—a disease associated with destitution. It was clearly established that in a long series of cases where patients had been removed to the workhouse within five or six days of the illness, whether from slum court dwellings or from cellars, no further cases followed, but in an equally long series in which the patient had been left at home, all the members of the family who had not already had the disease were infected.[1] The recurrence of the disease after sulphur fumigation of the room and disinfection of the clothes by dry heat was exceedingly rare.

With regard to smallpox, of which the public mind inherits a dread from pre-vaccination days, the evidence was equally cogent; one illustration is sufficient to show both the mischief resulting from a patient being left at home where the visits of sympathetic or curious friends in turn carry the disease, and also the multiplication of centres of infection producing the epidemic.

Activity of the Council was stimulated in 1885 by an outbreak of smallpox, and the Council to meet it rented some 15 acres of land at Dingle Point from the Dock Board, upon which structures of a very temporary nature were erected to accommodate 200 patients. These structures were replaced in later years by wooden buildings as the Mersey Docks and Harbour Board allowed the tenancy of the land to continue.

The next step was to take over and extend the Netherfield Road Hospital to 100 beds; adjoining streets were demolished in order to acquire the necessary land for this purpose. This was completed in 1887, and, it was hoped, would meet the needs of the north end of the city; an excellently planned hospital in Grafton Street with 80 beds was also completed in the same year, which it was thought would meet the needs of the south part of the city. But the rôle of the Hospital in the prevention of

[1] See p. 57.

disease was becoming more widely understood; when in 1895 the incorporation into the city of the adjoining townships in which its natural outgrowths had taken place was arranged, although some of these out-townships had small institutions, yet, in view of a more extensive scheme, in only one case, namely that of West Derby, was it found desirable to maintain and extend it. In 1898 the first step to give effect to the intentions of the Council by the purchase of the Harbreck Estate at Fazakerley, comprising 120 acres, largely through the efforts of Dr Thomas Clarke, then Chairman of the Hospitals Committee, enabled finality upon the hospital question to be reached. The decision to proceed with suitable hospital accommodation upon this site was acted upon, and in due course an adjoining 30 acres of land were purchased and the finely equipped buildings completed. Within the large area of the Fazakerley Estate provision was made on carefully considered lines for the treatment and isolation of all forms of infections, and also a large area set aside for tuberculous patients.[1] The Sparrow Hall section, intended for smallpox, lies about three-quarters of a mile to the north-east of that devoted to other infections. The Sanatorium, which lies east of the Infectious Diseases section, was approaching completion at the beginning of the War, and in its unfinished state was handed over to the military authorities for use in conjunction with the rest of the various establishments. During 1919 this section was restored to the Liverpool Corporation and the repairs necessary for the uses for which it was built were completed, giving accommodation for 250 patients.

It would be difficult to point to any example of necessary municipal expenditure in which benefits alike to the direct recipients and to the community are more strongly marked. Years of experience have amply confirmed the value of the Hospitals as the indispensable link in the chain of preventive medicine which they have proved to be. They have been an essential factor in the control and virtual disappearance of the infections for which they were originally provided, and a large section of their accommodation had for many years been utilised with equal usefulness in lessening forms of infection at one time regarded as minor.

[1] See p. 74.

It is obvious, however, that hospitals controlled by Sanitary Authorities must, from the nature of the cases dealt with, be subject to an administrative regime altogether different from that of general hospitals.

Although in cities of wide extent more than one is necessary, yet both economy and efficiency are met by extensive units in one area, and under one supervision, as at Fazakerley, rather than by scattered independent units, each involving its special administrative machinery and looked to, perhaps, to deal with every emergency case which may arise.

As elsewhere, so in the various county boroughs or townships abutting or forming part of the port of Liverpool, provision for cases of smallpox presents the most difficult problem; the question is not merely of local or even national importance, but has an international significance proportionate to the commercial ramifications of the port. Smallpox *in any part* of the area of one of these county boroughs or townships will have the same significance, from the Consular or shipping point of view, as it would within the defined area of the Port Sanitary Authority, so far as international agreements are concerned.[1]

Obviously, therefore, a close co-ordination between the various riparian authorities is necessary and in 1923, as the result of a conference specially convened for the purpose, it was felt that, although a single hospital for smallpox would be an ideal solution of the question, the difficulties of river transport made necessary the provision of one hospital available for the areas on the Liverpool side and one for the areas on the Birkenhead side of the Mersey; provisional adjustments on these lines were agreed to. In the event of any outbreak of threatened seriousness in any one area, advantages, it was felt, would accrue from an arrangement by which trained officers of another of the constituent authorities could, upon request, be concentrated upon the infected area.

[1] See p. 13.

Chapter V

ADMINISTRATIVE DEVELOPMENTS

District Nursing—Employment of Trained Nurses in the Poor Law Hospitals—The Universities and Public Health—Drs Parkes and Sanderson—Employment of Women in Health Administration—Health Visitors—Welfare of Mothers and Children—Milk Depots—Clinics—Valuable help from Voluntary Associations—Treatment of Ophthalmia—Midwives—Midwives Act—Midwives Association—National Insurance Act and Maternity Benefit—Female Staff during the War.

DISTRICT nursing, which now constitutes one of the most valuable social services of the country, originated in Liverpool in 1859, the endeavour being to provide the sick poor with some skilled nursing in their homes.

The movement was initiated by the late Mr W. Rathbone, who, prior to that date, had experienced the great benefit of skilled nursing at home in his own family and desired to extend it to the poor. He began in a tentative way with a single experiment. He persuaded Mrs Robinson, the nurse whose services inspired the idea, to undertake the work for three months at his expense; she was to attend the sick poor in their own homes, nurse them and teach them how to help themselves, and she was supplied with all necessaries for the purpose. There was no town in the country at that time where greater poverty and worse housing conditions prevailed than Liverpool, and Mrs Robinson encountered so much misery that at the end of a month she begged to be released from her engagement; but she was induced to continue by the argument that much of the evil she had seen might be prevented, and by the hope of preventing it. She persevered and found so much satisfaction in the real and certain good she was able to do that at the end of three months she begged to be allowed to devote herself entirely to the work instead of nursing the well-to-do. The results had, indeed, exceeded expectations; the timely and skilled care had not only restored the sick to health in several cases, but had had secondary effects of still greater value in giving to the family better ideals of living.

The success of the experiment led Mr Rathbone to seek its extension, but the difficulty was to find nurses. Nursing as a skilled profession was then still in its infancy, and there was little or no systematic teaching. Mr Rathbone sought the advice, among others, of Florence Nightingale, who had been trained in Germany, and whose work in the Crimea had given a great impetus to the nursing movement. The suggestion was made that nurses should be trained at the Liverpool Royal Infirmary, but there were no facilities for the purpose, and the Infirmary itself at that time appears to have had no really trained nurses on its staff. There was no accommodation for probationers or nurses.

It became a duty to continue and extend the work which had such a successful beginning. There was, fortunately, no doubt that the necessary funds would be forthcoming, but there was another drawback of a serious nature; the skilled nurses, without whom funds were useless, could nowhere be obtained. The only means, therefore, of supplying the demand for trained nurses was to form a school of nursing in Liverpool, the course suggested and recommended by Miss Nightingale.[1]

The authorities of the Royal Infirmary in Liverpool had already realised the want of such a school for infirmary and private nursing; as a step towards the improvement of the nursing standard the matron of that institution had been empowered to pay a salary of £16 to any nurse who deserved it; no more than four nurses were deemed worthy to receive it, and the ordinary nurse of that time, if paid more than the usual salary of £10, would most probably have incurred dismissal for drunkenness after the first quarter-day. The need was recognised and Mr Gibbon, the Chairman of the Royal Infirmary, favoured the idea and took the preliminary step of making a personal examination of the nursing organisation at King's College and St Thomas's Hospitals, London; lack of accommodation, however, proved the greatest obstacle to its fulfilment until Mr Rathbone, who had become a member of the Royal Infirmary Committee,

[1] William Rathbone, *Organisation of Nursing*, published 1865.

asked permission to provide the accommodation at his own expense; the proposal was accepted, and in this way the Liverpool Training School and Home for Nurses was brought into being in 1863. It was a modern building in the construction of which Mr Horner, the architect, was much indebted to the suggestions of Miss Nightingale, who gave the plans the same consideration as if (to use her own words) "she were herself going to be the matron". The school was of necessity dependent upon the infirmary, whose matron supervised the nurses.

Florence Nightingale, writing of the newly constructed Training School and Home and its organisation, says:

I have studied all the Rules and Forms with the greatest profit and interest to myself—as indicating a master hand in securing that unity yet independence of action, that personal responsibility and yet liberty, which are so vitally essential to the continuance and development of a great and wide charity like this.

If any argument were required on behalf of the training of nurses ...for district work...the best argument is the success which has attended the efforts made in Liverpool,...greater than even the most sanguine hopes could have foreseen....The work opens a new chapter...the example will spread to every town and district in the Kingdom if wisely inaugurated in Liverpool. So far as it has gone, it has proved its own future possibility by its past success, and promises to be one of the most important agencies for coping with human misery which the present day has put forth. Let us all wish it Godspeed.[1]

In a very short time eighteen nurses were at work in as many districts in Liverpool, an arrangement which gave the work its name. A lady superintendent was appointed in each district (that is to say a person whose compassion and local interests prompted her to the work and who undertook supervision of details of management). Medical men and officers of religion co-operated in this work, and the Liverpool Central Relief and Charity Organisation Society, which was formed about this time by the combination of several philanthropic bodies, agreed in certain cases to give necessities to patients under the charge of district nurses. Arrangements were also made with this

[1] Extracts from Florence Nightingale's Introduction to Mr William Rathbone's *Organisation of Nursing*, 1865, and *The Life of William Rathbone*, by Eleanor Rathbone, 1905.

Society by which patients likely to benefit by sea air and sea bathing were sent for three weeks' residence at Southport.

The value of the voluntary aspects of this work, as distinguished from the "mechanical charity" of parochial relief, is not overlooked in the numerous reports relating to it. An interesting side-light is thrown on this aspect of the work by the fact that

some have objected to allow the ladies of their family to take part in the work for fear of infection.... The nurse can always tell the Lady Superintendent where she may safely go, and can avoid visiting her on days when, or in clothes in which, she has attended infectious cases. But if the risk were greater than it is, we should have no right to flinch from it. Life was given not to be hoarded, but to be carefully and wisely spent.

Other great cities were following the example of Liverpool —Manchester and Salford in 1864, Leicester in 1867, London with the East London Nursing Society in 1868, Birmingham in 1870; and in more recent years expansions followed over the whole country.

In Liverpool in 1875 the district nurses, instead of occupying separate lodgings, were placed in a District Nurses Home in Eldon Place, and in subsequent years nursing homes were established in six separate districts by benevolent persons impressed by the claims of those whose misfortunes were due to circumstances beyond their individual control. It is unfortunately not possible in the limited space available to trace further developments in detail, but the work of district nursing, i.e. nursing the sick poor in their own homes by means of trained nurses working under an organised system, received a national sanction when the bulk of the sum presented to Her Majesty in the year 1887 on the occasion of her Jubilee was devoted to the work, and thereby made the undertaking a royal and national one. It was decided that a sum of £76,000 should be expended in founding a national institution for the education and maintenance of nurses, and two years later the Queen Victoria Jubilee Institute for nurses was constituted.

This change (i.e. the organisation of skilled nursing) is perhaps the best fruit the past half-century has to show.... Of all the forms that charity takes, there is hardly one that is so directly successful as district nursing. It is almost true to say that wherever a nurse enters, the standard of life is raised....[1]

The growth of the work prior to 1887 and the decision of the Queen, in that year, already alluded to, led Her Majesty to constitute the Queen Victoria Jubilee Institute with a President and Council to represent the interests of the work which was growing so rapidly all over the kingdom. Some apprehension was felt that the newly constituted Council might seek to interfere with the management of local work. Happily no desire to do this was evinced, and the position and the prestige of the Council were strengthened by the affiliation with Liverpool. The Liverpool Association and the Queen's Institute proved of mutual benefit to one another.

In 1897 the proceeds of the city fund collected to commemorate the Queen's long reign were devoted to the extension of the work; the amount collected during the Lord Mayoralty of Sir Thomas Hughes, amounting to £23,000, was augmented by the David Lewis Trustees by £10,000 for the building of a Central Home, the training facilities having long since been taken up by all of the great Liverpool hospitals.

It was through the instrumentality of Mr William Rathbone that a great reform by the system of employing trained nurses was introduced in 1865 in the Liverpool workhouse hospital under the supervision of Miss Agnes Jones, the then lady superintendent. The effort to give some training to the female paupers with the object of employing them as a kind of under-nurse wholly failed and the idea was abandoned. Agnes Jones fell a victim to typhus fever in 1868, but she had already achieved success in her pioneer work, and the system of employing trained nurses spread quickly to parish hospitals and to workhouse hospitals all over the country. It is beyond the scope of this volume to follow this interesting subject further, but the extension of the system throughout the country was an incalculable benefit to the sick poor in all Poor Law Institutions.

One word about maternity training, which, though everybody must be born, is at its very beginning. We mean by maternity

[1] Charles Booth, *Life and Labour*, final vol. p. 157.

training, teaching the care of the mother and infant after its birth, a most important branch which seems to be yet in its infancy, and a not very sanitary infancy it is.

Among the really initiated we hear the complaint that from even so-called "trained midwives", good *maternity practice*, especially in sanitary things, and in feeding the infant and teaching the mothers what to do, cannot be expected at the lying-in woman's own home. This, then, is not district nursing; and yet the midwife ought to be essentially the teacher and the district nurse of lyings-in at home.[1]

The Universities and Public Health

The City Council, dissatisfied with the slowness of progress, felt that the money expended had not achieved the expected results; it became discouraged and doubtful as to whether it was on the right path. Although there were occasional evidences that interest—not unstimulated by earlier severe visitations of cholera in the University towns themselves—in the subject of public health was not wholly dead in the English Universities, those centres of learning had not yet evolved any views helpful to the administrator, no doubt because they were not in a position to do so; they had never considered the matter. The first steps in the nature of an appeal, and that an indirect one, to the Universities was made by Liverpool in 1869, when the guidance of an outstanding scientist, Professor Huxley, was sought, and upon his advice Professor Burdon-Sanderson of Oxford, and Dr Parkes, the Professor of Hygiene in the Military School, were invited to report upon certain questions affecting the sanitation of the city.

Their report presented in 1871 proved a valuable one; an additional difficulty in the case of Liverpool is alluded to and provides the forecast of port and international hygiene which has been so remarkably developed in recent years. The following is the statement: "The introduction of typhus, cholera, smallpox, or relapsing fever is always attended with epidemic outbreaks, if the disease prevail in places with which it is in frequent communication as a seaport. It is not possible", they say, "to alter this without surrendering the commercial supremacy of Liverpool, but some precautionary measures may be taken."

[1] Extracts from Florence Nightingale's Introduction to Mr Rathbone's book.

Efforts, they suggest, should be made to obtain regular monthly reports of the health of foreign countries as regards epidemic diseases, so as to be prepared for any contingency of the kind.

"Drunkenness and the consequent poverty, degradation and squalor, lead", as the Report states, "to starvation and beggary. The children are in rags and filth, and the unhappy people seem to know none of the comforts, and few of the decencies of life, and widespread habits of drunkenness, and consequent want of food, aid their wretched homes in destroying their health."

About this period Sir Henry Acland, Regius Professor of Medicine at Oxford, had begun to take an active interest in hygiene, and it would seem largely owing to him that another Royal Commission had been appointed to inquire into the unsatisfactory condition of metropolitan and other drainage. William Stokes, Regius Professor of Medicine at Dublin, and a friend of Acland, was one of the earliest, ablest and most distinguished advocates of the doctrines of State medicine, and for many years used all his powers of mind, of eloquence and of learning to advance those doctrines. It was to him that the initiation of the teaching of the subject in Dublin University and the founding in 1872 of a diploma in State medicine in connection with Trinity College were mainly due. He says:

A time may come when the conqueror of disease will be more honoured than the victor in a hundred fights. The time may come when no man for his own ends or for his own profit will be permitted to damage the health or the well-being of his neighbour or of his servant, or his employee, nor the prisoner have to suffer through the ignorance or the indifference of his jailer....

The gifts to man from Heaven—pure air, pure water, bright light and wholesome food—will be more freely shared in, and the moral and physical evils of overcrowding and the consequent guilt, the shame and the pestilence will disappear.

In the University of Edinburgh certain aspects of the subject had been systematically dealt with at an earlier date, and to a fuller extent, than in any of the other Universities. The sequence of the teaching of the subject affords an interesting explanation of the association of the prevention of disease as a science with the science of medical jurisprudence. These subjects, to-day,

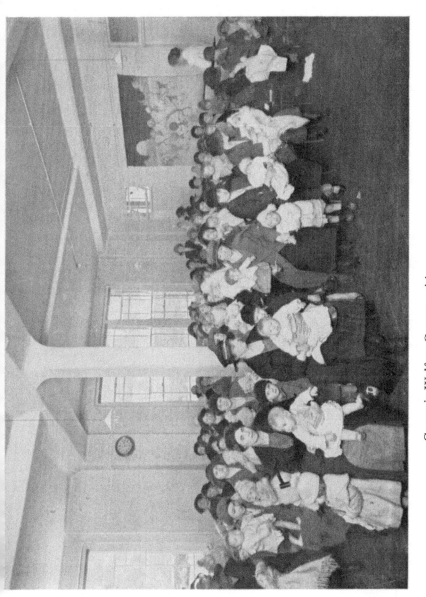

Carnegie Welfare Centre waiting-room.

are really as wide apart as the poles, but at that time the problems with which each was concerned had a common origin. Public health, as a science, crept into the Universities in the tracks of the medical jurist simply because conditions favouring disease were identical with those favouring the crimes which, at that time, mainly claimed the attention of the medical jurist. Public health problems, under the title of "Medical Policy", were included in Professor Traill's lectures at Edinburgh, before 1862, under various headings, for instance, prostitution, sewers, schools, effects of dwellings on health, climate, etc. His syllabus would appear to have been founded on French and German text-books of that day. "Medical policy" was considerably amplified by Sir Douglas Maclagan, but perhaps received its greatest stimulus and most practical application from Sir Henry Littlejohn, who was lecturing on the subject at the extra-mural school of medicine long before his appointment to the Chair of Medical Jurisprudence within the University. He was at that time the Medical Officer of Health of the city, and had availed himself of the exceptional opportunities to give practical instruction.

At the University of Glasgow Sir William Gairdner from 1862 had a large share in laying the foundations of the public health system of that city; further developments of the subject which ensued are due to Professor Glaister.

Once the subject had obtained a foothold, the Universities of Oxford and Cambridge were not slow to recognise that the health and well-being of the people were subjects worthy to be included in the scope of their attention, but it is clear that among the many difficulties which obstructed advance was the fact that the most appropriate lines of research and teaching had still to be found. Under the Public Health Act of 1872 every Sanitary Authority was required to appoint a Medical Officer of Health; this Act gave a powerful stimulus to the foundation of courses of systematic instruction, and in due time diplomas for special knowledge of the subject were granted—Dublin in 1872, Cambridge, largely through the interest of Dr Liveing, in 1874, and Edinburgh at the same time. At the University of Cambridge the subject was fostered under the influence of Mr Purvis, the late Sir Sims Woodhead, and others, and the course of instruction was largely attended. The diploma in Public Health, given under the State Medicine Syndicate, was a popular one, and its high standard has been fully recognised by administrative bodies. The University of London, in 1875, instituted an examination in subjects which related to public health, and awarded a certificate of proficiency in those subjects. In 1887 a movement was set on foot by the General Medical Council to standardise the qualifications issued by the various Universities. In June, 1888, public health was recognised in the University of London as a distinct branch of study and subject for examination, and the Senate established a degree in State medicine in place of the certificate in public health, to be awarded to Bachelors of Medicine. The Local Government Act of 1888, mainly at the instance of the Royal Institute of Public Health, required that a medical officer of health appointed after 1902 should be the registered holder of a diploma in public health.

When the University Colleges of Manchester, Liverpool, Leeds, Cardiff, Sheffield, and Birmingham raised themselves to University dignity—and for our present point of view Durham may be included—the importance of the subject of the health of the people had already received full recognition, and provision was made for the training of medical officers of health and their ancillary staffs, medical officers of schools, of welfare clinics, of tuberculosis and venereal disease clinics, and so forth. Similar provision was also made for city and county bacteriologists and analysts, and in some instances for the education of the general public, as for example at the Liverpool University School of Hygiene.

Nor was the training of the rank and file of the sanitary army yet so fully recognised. Knowledge which is the possession of a few can only benefit a few; just as in the monastic days of the older Universities the value of the trained itinerant preachers was recognised, so to-day the Universities, or some of them, recognise the vital importance of the training of those officers who are in daily touch with the people, and whose business it is to translate and apply established facts. Amongst this class are sanitary inspectors and health visitors, the staffs engaged in the inspection of meat and foodstuffs, or in the suppression of smoke and the proper control of boiler furnaces, and so forth. It is in connection with the University schools of social science, or public health, that this training is provided, and the certification of the candidate follows, as in the case of the diploma for the medical officer. Generous grants towards the cost of this training are made by the Ministry of Health.

It is clear that the policy of present-day health movements is increasingly directed to educational methods. It is with these objects that sanitary inspectors, welfare workers or health visitors are employed, that clinics are established, and that industrial employers safeguard their employees. "Health Weeks", "Baby Weeks", lectures, literature, models, exhibitions, all help to create an educated public opinion, and we all of us appreciate the services of the statesman, cleric, or popular actor or actress who is good enough, on occasion, to convey to the public the homely truths, which are so much more arresting when coming through these channels rather than through the usual ones.

While there is no need to fear that the Universities are likely to slacken in their interest, one need only study the writings of Chadwick, Simon, J. B. Russell, or many others, to find, as one might expect, that the influences of the Government to encourage or discourage their efforts are very potent.

Professors Parkes and Sanderson

The references made by the Council in November 1870 to Professors Parkes and Burdon-Sanderson were specific in their nature, and comprised points which now would be regarded as the merest elementary principles of sanitation, but the fact is indicative of the rudimentary development of sanitary knowledge in this country.

Their Report to the Council recommended that dirty stagnant ponds and unsightly pits should be filled up by builders' refuse only, and that no building should be erected upon any other deposit for at least two years from the date of the last. They make the curious recommendation that:

It should be inquired also whether some system of sorting could not be resorted to and the more offensive matters picked out. It might be possible to employ the paupers in the Workhouse for the purpose, or to authorise small payments to the persons who now make a living by raking over the cinders after deposit, for such vegetable and animal refuse as they can pick out. Of course any such sorting would have to be done under some kind of supervision.

They thought it advisable to exclude the introduction of chemical refuse into sewers from which gas might be evolved, and they allude to the defective condition of drains in

The parts of the town where the houses are inhabited by persons of superior circumstances, and beyond the reach of official inspection, ...as the prevention of...this condition is beyond the control of the local authority, and efforts must be directed to keep those drains which are under their own management in such condition as to render the defects of private drains as little dangerous as possible.

The state of the sewers as regards deposit was a matter which attracted their attention, and the associated deficiency of water for flushing receives emphasis. "This trouble", declared Mr Newlands, "had called for attention for many years"; twenty years previously he had recommended a plan for expeditious flushing and for washing the surface of streets and courts, and for allowing water to run freely along the channels for a certain time each day, to wash away all impurities, and in 1866 he had remarked that "our water supply has never been in a condition to admit of this. The deficient water supply has thrown us back after 18 years to much the same condition in which we were in 1848, with the difference of extended works and increased wants".

On the question about the modification of the proposals regarding the water carriage system, they say "it would be useless for us to enter into argument against the return to the barbarous system of middens", and they recommend the extension of water carriage and its application to the town as a whole.

In the second part of their Report they say "the ordinary annual mortality in years not marked by any great epidemic disease is about 35 per 1000. In the years with epidemic outbreaks of Typhus, Cholera, or diseases of that class, it may even amount to 50 per 1000". Having regard to the position of Liverpool as a seaport the introduction of typhus, cholera, or smallpox they regard as certain if these diseases prevail in places with which it is in communication. Then follows the curious statement, "it is not possible to alter this without surrendering the commercial supremacy of Liverpool, but some precautionary measures may be taken".

Various streets are contrasted in regard to mortality rates, and the astonishing fact emerges that in Sawney Pope Street the infant mortality rate was approximately 398 per 1000, a rate which had persisted for the four preceding years.

The inferences drawn from this excessive infant mortality are:

That a large number of deaths from the contagious diseases of childhood must be expected in a crowded population where removal and isolation are impossible. But...from this table alone, it might be confidently predicted that the people, among whom such a high death rate occurs from these causes, are not only poor, but are careless, ignorant, and probably barbarous in their modes of life....

...The great death rate of Liverpool in non-epidemic years is therefore in some measure owing to the great mortality of children.

But in addition to this, we found the floor of the cellars, in several cases, in a very foul condition. Impurities of all kinds had been deposited there, and in this way the air of the house was constantly contaminated from the basement.

When we visited these courts at night, it was singular how pure even the air of the courts appeared after coming out of the almost insupportable fœtor of the sleeping rooms. We ought to state that we visited these courts during cold weather, when windows are less frequently opened than in summer.

With regard to the people and furniture in these houses, we were not at all prepared either for the wretched appearance of the people, or for the terrible aspect of poverty disclosed. All this is so familiar to the Town Council and to the Officers of Health, that we feel we are going over ground too well known. But it is necessary to the completeness of our sketch to state, that we could not have believed that in any town in this country we could have gone into room after room, and house after house, and have found in so many cases literally almost nothing but the bare walls, a heap of straw covered by dirty rags, and possibly the remainder of a broken chair or table.

We were much struck by two circumstances in these houses, in addition to the want of furniture. There were no cooking utensils of any kind, or only an old saucepan. The inmates thus depended for the means of rudely cooking what food they could get (in our visits chiefly fish and bread) on a neighbour's kindness. The second point was that it was evident many persons had no change of clothes. On pressing the inquiry as to how they washed, and what they did at night, we extracted from several that they occasionally washed their hands and faces at the tap, but seldom removed their clothes. In some cases, both of men and women, we made out that the clothes had not been removed for several weeks. In our visits at night, we sometimes found that the clothes had been partly removed, and were then drawn over the person. Some men, indeed, were in bed quite naked, lying on the straw and covered with their clothes.

The impression made upon us by these circumstances has been so deep, that we may unconsciously exaggerate their frequency. It must be remembered that we are referring only to the worst parts of the town, and we should be sorry to apply this description to the houses of the mass of the labouring population in Liverpool. But certainly we can safely say, that the relative number of these houses, and of the people living under these conditions, is much greater in Liverpool than in other towns of which we have knowledge.

With regard to the causes of this condition of the people, all to whom we have spoken attribute it to three circumstances: the irregularity of the labour market, the improvidence and careless habits of the people, and the great intemperance....

On this last point we are aware that numerous investigations have been made in Liverpool, and that no additional evidence is needed from us. But following our course of independent inquiry, we endeavoured to make out what part intemperance played in producing this poverty, and all its attendant evils. We cannot doubt that it plays a very large part.

When the occupation is uncertain, like that of a dockyard labourer, the case is nearly the same; the temperance which is enforced from time to time by destitution, is compensated for at the first opportunity on the return of plenty.

It does not appear that the bad trade of the last few years has lessened the amount of drinking; all agreed that there is much more than formerly.

...The unhappy people seem to know none of the comforts and few of the decencies of life, and widespread habits of drunkenness, and consequent want of food, aid their wretched homes in destroying their health.

In recommending the construction of new streets it was pointed out that the powers vested in the Corporation were wholly inadequate for the purpose, and application to Parliament would be necessary.

Maternity and Child Welfare

As in other directions, so in the case of the welfare of children, voluntary effort has frequently paved the way for organised municipal procedure. Voluntarily supported day nurseries furnish an early instance, the object being to care for very young children while the mother was at work; the "Adam Cliff" Nursery, 63 Everton Road, opened in 1874, appears to have been the first, followed by others under the aegis of the Liverpool Ladies Sanitary Association and other voluntary bodies. Their sphere of usefulness was in due course extended by training young women as nursery nurses, and they later proved helpful in training Health Visitors.

The adverse conditions of domestic life in the lower quarters of the city, already described, led in the early 'nineties to the conviction that valuable results would follow the employment of suitably qualified women, if such could be found, for the purpose of visiting the houses and advising the occupants. The suggestion was regarded as impracticable and at first met with no support, indeed it was humorously suggested that the employment of 10,000 charwomen to clean the homes in question would be more to the point. However, in 1897, as an experiment, two women were added to the sanitary staff for the purpose indicated; this marked an initial step in a movement which ultimately spread to all Sanitary Authorities and in later years received the warm support of the Government; Miss Radcliffe, one of those appointed, had been associated with the Society for the Prevention of Cruelty to Children almost from its inception in Liverpool in 1883.[1] The occupation of the other, Miss Burton, had been more or less of an educational and business nature.

Their services proved so useful that in 1899 six more appointments were made, and the number was gradually added to in succeeding years as their value became recognised. Just as there were difficulties to be overcome in making provision for the training of nurses for district and hospital work, so there were difficulties to be overcome in providing the means of training for those desirous of taking up public health work in the capacity of health visitors or inspectors. The need was ultimately met by the

---

[1] See pp. 41, 106.

establishment of the University School of Hygiene, which was rendered possible by the co-operation of the City Council with the University, assisted by the generosity of Lord Leverhulme, members of the Holt family, the late Mr John Rankin, and many others. As candidates became attracted to posts of this kind increased facilities for affording them the necessary instruction were provided by the Sanitary Science Instruction Committee of the University School of Hygiene, in conjunction first with the Liverpool Ladies Sanitary Association (founded in 1891) and subsequently with the University School of Social Science, and the Board of Education espoused and contributed to the cost of the scheme. In due course candidates were required to give evidence by certificate of efficient training, for which the best groundwork was found to be the three years' training provided for nurses in approved hospitals. When in later years the functions exercised by the Board of Education were taken over by the Ministry of Health, the grants in aid were continued but the granting of certificates of qualification was limited to a board of examiners in London which was unfamiliar with the problems of actual teaching and prescribed a course of training unnecessarily long and too costly to be practicable, occasioning, until it was modified, a shortage of desirable candidates.

In 1901 the Health Committee made contributory grants to various voluntary centres, and in this year, in view of the continued high infant mortality in the lower quarters of the city, largely the result of improper feeding, followed the example set by Dr Budin in 1892 in his "Goutte de Lait" enterprises in France, and took the highly important step of establishing depots for the supply of milk specially adapted to the needs of infants of various ages whose mothers were not able to suckle them. Many difficulties had, however, to be overcome; the necessary plant had to be devised as no firm existed which made a plant of the kind. The work was necessarily experimental and many modifications were made before success was achieved.

Dr Budin had established his cliniques in Paris in connection with the obstetrical service; in that city as a whole the infant mortality from 1897 to 1901 amounted to 178 per 1000, the infant loss amongst those attending his "Clinique" and "Consultation de Nourrissons" during the same period was only

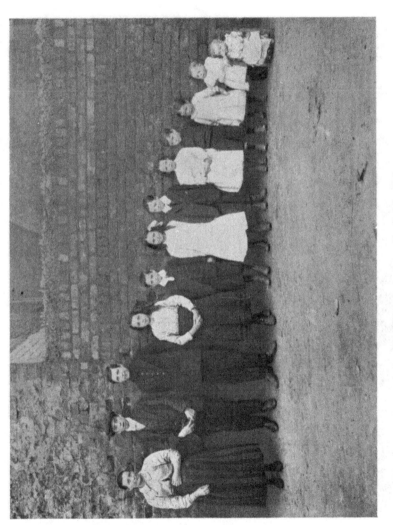

A family of eleven naturally fed in infancy.

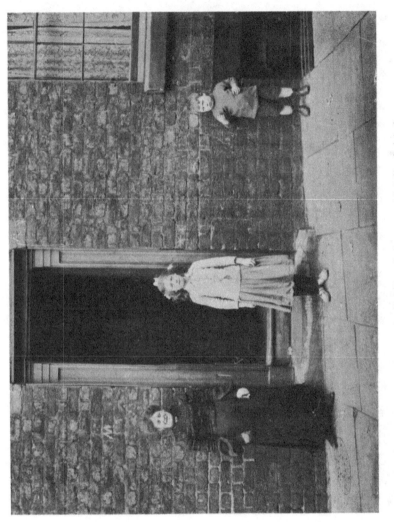

Two survivors of a family of eleven artificially-fed infants.

46 per 1000. From Paris the "Consultation de Nourrissons" or "Gouttes de Lait" radiated all over France—the forerunners of the welfare centres and ante-natal and post-natal clinics of this country.

The complete substitute for the milk of a healthy mother will never be found, as the infant grows the quality of the mother's milk varies to adapt it to the infant's needs, niceties in Nature which no laboratory can imitate. When recourse must be had to artificial feeding, cow's milk sterilised and of good quality was used by Budin, Variot and Dufour for many years. The prejudice against it in this country rested on apprehensions of infantile scurvy, but happily experience dispelled these apprehensions in France as it did in due course in England.

At the French cliniques the progress of infants was gauged by periodic weighing, a procedure which many Liverpool mothers at first regarded as "unlucky". But the undertaking received support from the medical profession, and an especially hearty co-operation from the staff of the Children's Infirmary. The Corporation, in fact, had been successful in the rôle of foster-mother for infants who could not be suckled by their mothers; the evidence of medical men, and of personal observations, all pointed to the saving of child life by this method.

By the year 1913, of some 25,000 infants who had been fed by this artificial food 17,547 were supplied through the depots, and the remainder through dairies; it was possible to keep very careful observation on the former. Many of the infants were extremely ill, perhaps hopelessly ill, at the time when they were brought to the depots, and generally the conditions of health were below the normal, but amongst them the mortality was 88 per 1000, contrasting favourably with the mortality of 138 per 1000 in the rest of the city.

What these infants would have been fed on, and with what result, if it were not for the provision so made, may be imagined. Even when suitable food for the infant was handed over in proper condition to the mother, much home visiting, watching and guidance were necessary to ensure its proper use.[1]

[1] The illustrations between pages 104 and 105 illustrate two families under the same social conditions in each of which 11 children were born. In the first case all the infants were suckled and survived, in the second artificial feeding was adopted and 9 died in infancy.

During the year 1913 dried milk, very much cheaper to use, was coming into use. The difficulty, however, was the inability of many mothers to understand how to mix the food properly, or to protect it from contamination.

At this time Professor Beattie and Dr Lewis, of the Liverpool University Laboratories, were conducting a long series of investigations into promising and important methods of sterilisation of milk by electricity. Their results proved wholly successful, but it was not possible to overcome certain difficulties in their application to public usefulness, and this valuable agency has remained in abeyance.

The milk depots eventually developed into the establishment of the civic ante- and post-natal clinics and welfare centres; grants in aid were continued to voluntary organisations, or they were taken over and extended by the Corporation.

Medical officers were assigned to these centres and they were increasingly availed of by the people. Sir Arthur Newsholme[1] remarks that the value of the centre depends chiefly on the medical service given in it. Professor Budin's view is "An infant consultation is worth precisely as much as the presiding physician". This is even more true for the ante-natal work of the centre, but its value is enhanced by the staff of health visitors and the encouragement and incentive to the mother, who appreciates the fact that others, like herself, value the health of her child.

In 1914 a very comprehensive scheme was in operation and the Local Government Board contributed one-half the entire cost of undertakings carried on under the aegis of the City Council, and a similar sum through the Health Committee to approved voluntary associations working in co-ordination with the Public Health Authorities of the city. The aim was to meet the necessities of the expectant mothers and provide subsequently for the care of the mother and infant.

Meanwhile the painstaking and patient operations of the Society for the Prevention of Cruelty to Children (originated under the leadership of the late Mr Agnew, the Manager of the Liverpool branch of the Bank of England) were bearing good fruit. Its efforts, supplemented by legislation, local or general,

---

[1] *Local Government Board Report on Maternity and Child Welfare*, 1916.

and notably by the Children Act of 1908, and by the sympathetic co-operation of the police, had effected a great change in the treatment of children. Intemperance, the great source of cruelty to children, was diminishing and cases of aggressive cruelty were becoming far less frequent. The efforts of the Society so changed the complexion of affairs that it was gradually becoming a Society for promoting the general welfare of children rather than one merely of guardianship from violence. Among its numerous activities the Society, in conjunction with the Health Committee, provided fire-guards for the use of poor families who, owing to lack of means, found difficulty in buying them.

In 1905 an agency viewing children from quite another aspect was inaugurated. In that year the Society for the Care of Invalid Children (now the Child Welfare Association) was initiated under the inspiring leadership of Miss Margaret Beavan as an independent endeavour to ensure that invalid children should be taken to suitable institutions, and that the necessary home care, whether of children leaving hospitals or of those who were or had been attending as out-patients, should be continued. The Education Committee appreciated the value of the work and the Association became the Care Committee of the Liverpool Education Committee's special schools for defective children, and secured cots at the West Kirby Convalescent Home for their treatment. Co-operation with the Health Department was early ensured and some of the city hospitals promptly aided in making provision for the further care of children leaving the hospitals.

In 1913 a much-needed hospital for children suffering from surgical tuberculosis was founded by the Child Welfare Association at Leasowe. A Treasury grant of £17,000 towards the hospital was received and the total amount subsequently spent on the hospital amounted to £150,000.

Under the complete scheme for dealing with tuberculosis which had been drawn up by the Medical Officer of Health, and approved by the City Council, the maintenance grants, which were issued to any hospital dealing with this subject, were received by the Leasowe Hospital. These grants were made jointly by the Insurance Committee, the Local Government Board, the City Council, and later by the Ministry of Health.

In 1914 the first hundred beds in the Leasowe Hospital were opened by Lord Derby, who had shown the great and helpful interest in the hospital which has characterised his association with all undertakings designed to improve the social welfare of the city.

In 1916 temporary provision was made at Leasowe for a much-needed hospital for babies. This work was transferred later (in 1924) to a more appropriate place at Woolton, a large privately occupied mansion being altered and largely extended, and this is now the Royal Liverpool Babies Hospital. It was visited by Her Majesty the Queen in 1927.

It is not possible in this volume to trace the different stages of administrative development in regard to the provision for the health of mothers and children, but the co-operation with voluntary effort has been a marked feature, the bulk of the work and cost falling on the municipal side, and the reward has been found in the remarkable saving of infant life and in the diminution of the avoidable adverse contingencies incidental to child-birth.

In 1916 the Carnegie United Kingdom Trust[1] devoted special attention to the physical welfare of mothers and children and a report upon the subject presented to them in 1917 led to a gift by the Trust of £25,000 for the establishment in Liverpool of a model welfare centre for mothers and infants. This centre, which was opened by Miss Haldane in December, 1923, and officially taken over by the Liverpool Corporation, has exerted a most beneficial influence in the directions for which it was established and has contributed its full share in the amelioration of conditions incidental to the welfare of mothers and children and the saving of infant life.[2]

The observation ward of the Carnegie Centre fulfils an extremely important function in that it receives infants whose ailments are obscure but who cannot safely be left at home, and who are not ill enough for admission to hospital, and in certain emergencies foster mothers have been found for infants through

---

[1] *Report of the Carnegie United Kingdom Trust on the Physical Welfare of Mothers and Children*, Part. I, by E. W. Hope, M.D., Part II, by Dame Janet Campbell, England and Wales, 1917.

[2] See chart.

the agency of the Maternity Hospital or the Quarry Bank Maternity Home and other sources. One of the general hospitals provides beds in its convalescent branch to which ante-natal patients may be sent on account of general ill-health.

At the Quarry Bank Maternity Home, which was opened in 1920, there have been 1524 confinements without any maternal deaths or puerperal sepsis. A weekly ante-natal clinic was commenced shortly after the opening, and the premises are soon to be extended.

After a few years' experience it was manifest that the health visitors were filling a highly important part on the sanitary staff, the many problems of infant life bringing them into close association with the work of the rapidly extending welfare centres and milk depots. The duties assigned to this important section of the staff, whilst varying from time to time, have grown steadily in responsibility; they include the visitation of neglected homes, attendance in the schools during the medical inspection of school children with a view to ensure that the necessary curative attention is given to those who require it. The school teachers co-operate with the health visitors and call their attention to any neglected, verminous, or filthy children attending school—the neglected child always proving a short cut to the neglected home.

The Police Aided Clothing Association, formed by the late Alderman Watts in 1895, was designed to clothe the numbers of neglected, dirty, ragged and shoeless or half-naked children, many of tender age, begging in the streets in all weathers, a spectacle which arrested the attention and excited the wonder of any visitor unfamiliar with it. The "police aid" ensured that the clothing given to the children should not be taken from them and pawned by the parents for drink, all articles being stamped and pawnbrokers duly apprised.

The health visitors attend the welfare centres and clinics and visit houses at which births are reported under the Notification of Births Act, 1908, to co-operate with the midwife as may be necessary.[1] Cards of instructions are left in these cases and any children found suffering from minor ailments are duly cared

[1] See p. 113.

for. Thus the health visitors have been able to co-operate in the great work. In many directions their services have been useful to the District Nursing Association, the Central Relief Committee and the relieving officers of the Boards of Guardians, and their inquiries assist the Housing Committee in ensuring that tenants in the re-constructed areas shall be selected from those dispossessed from their dwellings on sanitary grounds. Difficulties with language in the case of foreign Jews were met by the appointment of a health visitor familiar with Yiddish.

Special visitors are assigned to duties in connection with measles and whooping-cough, and also in the supervision of workshops in which women are employed.

The need for promptitude of treatment in ophthalmia neonatorum—inflammation of the eyes of the newly born—was met upon the initiative of Miss Elizabeth Rathbone in 1907 by two health visitors specially trained at St Paul's Eye Hospital being appointed by the Health Committee, and a ward in St Paul's Hospital set aside for babies suffering from that disease. It is an interesting commentary that when the infants were accompanied by their mothers recovery was very much more rapid than when the sufferers were admitted without them.

The needs of the unmarried mother and her baby have been met as in the case of others, and the prejudiced rule which excluded the unmarried mother from the benefits of the Maternity Hospital happily fell into disuse and disappeared from the regulations of that institution.

A source of mischief which exacted its toll from infant life, and which was revealed year after year in the coroner's court, was the suffocation of infants whilst in bed with their mothers; this usually occurred on a Saturday night and there were strong reasons to associate the disaster, happily a diminishing one, with inebriety. During 1890, for example, 165 inquests were held on infants who had met their death in this way. In 1929 the number was reduced to two.

In 1900 the writer pointed out that the necessity for additional powers to ensure the more effectual protection of infants and young children whilst in the custody of drunken persons must sooner or later force itself upon public attention. Legislative powers to protect infants and young children were provided in the Children Act, 1908, an Act whose comprehensive provisions made child-life happier in many directions.

The committee which controls these diverse branches of work (see diagram, page 115) was originally designated the Infant Mortality Sub-Committee. The name was changed in 1906 to the Infant Life Preservation Committee and subsequently again altered to its more comprehensive title of Maternity and Child Welfare Committee, each succeeding title indicating more closely the objects the committee had in view and the comprehensive nature of its work.

The growth of the activities organised by the Health Committee and by voluntary associations, such as the Maternity Hospital, Royal Infirmary, or the Child Welfare Association, for the welfare of mothers, infants, and young children, and their appreciation by the public, is illustrated by the fact that the twenty-eight pre-maternity clinics had a total attendance of 10,766 during the year 1928. A large number of these cases are sent by medical practitioners, midwives, and health visitors, or by friends who have themselves benefited. The attendance at the post-natal clinics, both for mothers and infants, is also large. At the Carnegie Centre alone the attendance was 5618 in the same year.

The Women's Service Bureau, Gambier Terrace, under the direction of Miss Jessie Beavan, is a valuable organisation for the provision of clothing for the very poor mothers, and also for providing "home helps", that is women who can take the place of the housewife and attend to the children in the case of women confined at their own homes and who have no women relatives to assist them.

It has probably always been the case in Liverpool, as elsewhere, that the larger proportion of births have been attended by midwives. In Liverpool not less than 75 per cent. of the births are so attended, medical aid being called in only in the event of some emergency arising.

In 1895 the midwives were encouraged to form themselves into an association, as it is obviously easier to effect co-operation with an association than with the individuals who compose it, and such an association would foster a desire amongst themselves to observe any special rules or instructions to which their attention might be called.

At an early date the Midwives Association proved a valuable factor in the work of the various clinics, and notably in regard to the ante-natal clinics, in connection with which the midwives acted in close co-operation with the staff of health visitors. The Midwives Act of 1902 greatly facilitated this good relationship and directed more attention to the need for ante-natal care.

It was fortunate that training facilities for midwives had existed in Liverpool for so long, but the need for the better training of *all* women who undertook the practice of a midwife was gradually being felt all over the country, and legislation took the form of the Midwives Act of 1902.

The object of the Act was to secure better training for midwives and regulation of their practice under a Central Midwives Board. Giving three years' grace prior to its application, it provided that from April 1, 1905, no woman should use the title of midwife, or practise midwifery, unless she was certified under this Act, and no woman should be certified under this Act until she had complied with the rules and regulations laid down under the Act.

The rules of the Central Midwives Board prescribed a specified course of training, an examination, and subsequent certification of the midwife.

One obligation of the Act was that the midwife should call in medical aid in any abnormality affecting either the mother or the infant; no provision was made for the payment of the fee to a doctor for such service, usually rendered at night time; the Health Committee supplied the omission in the Act by guaranteeing suitable payment. Further, in view of the difficulties in poorer districts, where doctors were few, an arrangement was made with the Head Constable by which a telephone message would be sent by the police, from the nearest police station, to doctors who had expressed their willingness to take part in the scheme. The policemen on the beats would co-operate.

In 1905, when the Act came into operation, there were 361 midwives whose names had been inserted on the register, 305 of whom possessed qualifying certificates, the remaining 56, who had no certificates, had been in *bona fide* practice prior to July 31, 1901, and their names were also added to the register. The work of the midwives was supervised by a qualified officer appointed by the Medical Officer of Health to take note of their method of conducting their practice.

The midwives were now working in close co-operation with the Health Department and were prompt in calling the attention of the Department to any circumstances in the home which required its help.

The National Insurance Act, which came into operation during 1912, contained an important provision in regard to maternity benefit, namely, payment of a sum of forty shillings in the case of the confinement of the wife, or where the child is a posthumous child of the widow of an insured person, or of any other woman who is an insured person. This benefit is payable without reference to the legitimacy or otherwise of the child; the Insurance Acts have undergone various amendments and additions, but the 1924 Act renews this benefit among others relating to sickness and disablement. The wide activities of the National Insurance Committee, which radiate beneficially in all directions where the health and welfare of the people are concerned, are beyond the scope of the present subject.

In 1918 a further Midwives Act was passed which strengthened and amplified the powers of the Central Midwives Board, and made provision for the payment of medical practitioners who render emergency aid to midwives, thus extending to the whole country a procedure which had been in practice in Liverpool since 1904.

Throughout the War period the members of the Midwives Association were particularly helpful in their suggestions to prospective mothers, aiding their attendance at the ante-natal clinics, and themselves giving close attention to the domestic arrangements and their fitness or otherwise for the purposes of childbirth; at all times they have afforded much valuable help to the Health Department, of which indeed they might be regarded as an integral part. By this time they were all of them with few exceptions fully trained women, and the Association which they had been encouraged to form became numerically stronger, embracing practically all the midwives in the city. As an association they were able to, and did, arrange for themselves special courses of further instruction, in which they received much help in the way of lectures and so forth from the teachers

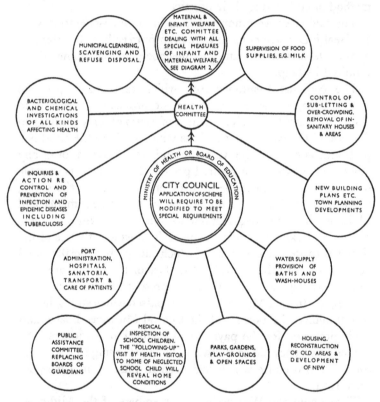

Diagram 1. Scheme of general sanitary administration and of allocation of duties to various committees.
Note. The National Insurance Committee, with wide ameliorative functions, is not a Committee of the Council.

of gynaecology in the University and from the gynaecologists of the city.

During the War the depletion of the male staff of the Public Health Department for military duty led to additions to the female staff; the marked decline in the number of births during this period lessened the calls of infancy, but the work of the department was greatly added to by special duties associated with the supply and rationing of food; cards of instructions drawn up by the Medical Officer and widely distributed, explained how restrictions of supplies in some directions could be

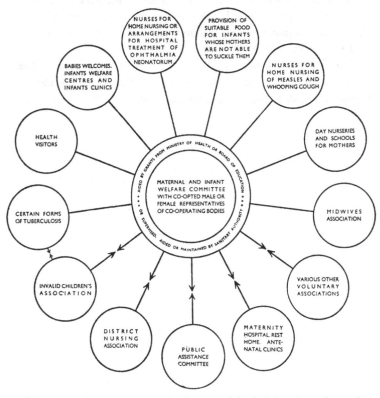

Diagram 2. Component agencies in a special administrative scheme for the promotion of maternal, infant and child welfare up to five years of age.

Note. The direct connecting lines between circles indicate official relationship. The arrows between circles indicate voluntary relationship.

more or less compensated by amplification in others. Full employment with liberal wages, in munition-making and other war-time occupations, removed the poverty incidental to precarious employment, and a sufficient food supply was within the reach of practically everybody. Food rationing involved many inconveniences and difficulties but rarely real hardship. Among other duties in which the staff took part were the visits to homes from which applications for relief had been received by the Prince of Wales Fund and Soldiers and Sailors Fund, and when, at the outbreak of war, with universal concurrence, the Fazakerley Hospital and others were handed over to the military authorities for the sick and wounded, the staff co-operated in the relief of the civilian occupants who uncomplainingly gave up their beds and were sent back to their homes.

The "ring" diagrams (pp. 114, 115) show at a glance the relationship and influence of the official and voluntary factors co-operating in an administrative scheme.

Chapter VI

SCHOOLS AND SCHOOL CHILDREN

Common Day Schools in the Early Days—Financial grants and school closure—Employment of Children Acts—Care of Defective Children—Provision of Meals—Medical Inspection of school children—Objects—Method—Parliamentary powers—Treatment—School Clinics—Advantageous co-operation—Causation of crippling in children—Defects arising during pre-school age—Comprehensive summary.

Common Day Schools in the Early Days

THE earlier accounts of the general state of the city afford a glance at the commencing educational efforts among the poorer classes and the condition of the common day and "dame" schools to which the children were sent. Mr Riddall Wood, who was a contemporary of Dr Duncan and specially interested in the subject, describes these schools in his evidence before the Royal Commission appointed to report upon the state of large towns in 1844–5. He referred to the schools in Liverpool, "in districts occupied by the humbler classes of people", as "most of them private adventure affairs injurious to the health of the children, in fact they appear to correspond with the conditions of the dwellings, wretched in the extreme, corresponding in a remarkable manner with the population....They are dark, damp, and dirty, used as dwelling, dormitory, and schoolroom, by the teacher's family". About forty of the "dame schools" in Liverpool were in cellars, many in garrets.

"Of the common day schools in the poorer districts of Liverpool it is difficult to convey an adequate idea, so close and offensive was the atmosphere in many of them as to be intolerable to a person entering from the open air." Animals were sometimes kept in the schoolrooms and Mr Wood alludes to one garret, 10 feet by 9, where a large number of children were found, the room being also occupied by poultry and three dogs, their noise drowning the voice of the teacher. The dimensions of the common day schoolroom rarely exceeded those of the "dame schools", whilst frequently the number of scholars was more than double. "I pointed out to the mistress of a 'dame school' that the state of things was injurious to the health of the children of the working class, to which she replied, 'They thrive best in dirt'".[1]

Mr Riddall Wood remarks that "the unwholesomeness is proved by the rapid spread of infections. The measles, scarlet fever, smallpox, and ophthalmic infections, never attack one scholar alone but frequently half of the scholars are affected at the same time, and some of the schools have been visited at times when two-thirds of the children usually attending were detained at home by such complaints".

(Question 2193) "You are aware in schools even of a superior class that unless the children are dispersed at once it runs through the school?" "Yes, but it occurs to me that it acquires greater virulence in the case of these schools." The question suggests the trend of common opinion of that time, the answer shows the closeness and accuracy of Mr Wood's observations.

Continuing his evidence he states that:

The Norfolk Street Boys' School is a large loft over a cowshed in a dirty and ill-ventilated back lane. No provision is made for girls in consequence of the want of funds to procure the necessary departments. The greater proportion of the children of these schools [a long list is given] were without shoes or stockings, or the common comforts of clothing, and yet attended even in the midst of winter in a half-naked and destitute condition.

I do not recollect a single instance of a school for the children of the working class having a playground or anything which would be considered of that character.

He stated that there were 30,000 children between the ages of 5 and 15 receiving no education, or who at all events did not appear to be attending any school.

This circumstance is commented on up to the passing of the Elementary Education Act of 1870. In 1868 Dr Trench observed that "one—and the most melancholy—feature in the condition of so many of the children of the poor of Liverpool is that they are entirely without occupation, without instruction, and mere

[1] Evidence before the Select Committee of the Royal Commission on the Health of Towns, 1844, Question 2189.

vagabonds in the streets. In no town of the kingdom is a compulsory education, if practicable, more required ".[1]

Elementary Education

Voluntary effort had long preceded the provision of schools out of funds compulsorily collected under the Education Act of 1870, particularly in the case of those whose infirmities or disabilities most needed help, for example, the school for teaching blind children, established in Liverpool as long ago as 1791, was the first institution of its kind in this or any other country. The Blue Coat School—Liverpool's oldest charity— the Seamen's Orphanage, and the orphan asylums, evidenced that care was taken of those whose claims were arresting.[2]

It is not less interesting and not less surprising to learn that when the Act of 1870 came into operation, Liverpool was officially reported to be one of the few large towns in which the provision which had been made by voluntary effort was considered to be equal to the estimated requirements. Presumably this related merely to the numerical estimate of the number of school "places", which indeed showed an actual excess of some 500 over the estimated requirement of 7500 in the parish, which appears to have arisen from the steady movement of the population outwards as areas of congested dwellings gave place to commercial premises and rendered some of the provision useless as it was then in the wrong place; the operations of the Liverpool Educational Aid Society had already been most helpful, as it paid the school fees of more then 4000 poor children; voluntary effort had also commenced to bridge the gap between elementary and secondary education by the provision of free scholarships which assisted a few promising scholars to pass from the elementary to the secondary schools. The standard of school accommodation improved with the standard of housing.

The Liverpool School Board constituted in 1870 was greatly aided a few years later by two voluntary associations, namely the Council of Education formed in 1874, and the Conference of School Managers established in 1875 to secure uniformity of

[1] *City Health Report*, 1868.
[2] See also index, Voluntary Associations.

action amongst the managers of elementary schools. In 1876 the School Board was led to establish classes for the teaching of pupil-teachers by the success of similar classes established in Liverpool by the Sisters of Notre-Dame.

The Technical Instruction Act of 1889 resulted *inter alia* in the appointment in 1897 of a Technical Sub-Committee of the Council with co-opted members representing the higher educational interests. The much-needed development of existing institutions was greatly aided and specific attention directed to the establishment of centres of special instruction; and a stimulus was given to the School of Hygiene and Sanitary Science, which had, like many other undertakings, been struggling with difficulties for many years.

Infectious Disease in Schools

In order to lessen the frequency with which schools became "exchanges" of infection, arrangements were made with the School Board by which the Medical Officer of Health was informed of children whose absence was due to illness, and suitable action was taken; conversely, when infectious sickness was found in a home from which children were in attendance at school, a notice was sent to the School Board and to the head teacher to exclude those children for a prescribed period.

At that time, infection of which the incidence is virtually limited to children, and to which outbreaks in the schools were commonly due, was lightly regarded; and in the absence of organisation and with very limited hospital accommodation other than the workhouse, children were left in their homes not unusually without medical aid until the disease, measles or whooping-cough for example, assumed a grave form. Meanwhile other children from the infected house, possibly themselves incubating the disease, were going to school, where their presence would infect others.

In 1890 the Infectious Diseases (Notification) Act, 1889, came into operation, and the interchange of information became more prompt and complete. The Act did not then include the notification of several important diseases, measles and whooping-cough for example, but nevertheless it paved the way for an amplification of the method already alluded to. As the organised co-operation of the staff of the Health Department with school attendance officers, head teachers, and principals of schools, became closer, the system was advantageously extended to all forms of infection, whilst a readier public appreciation of their value led, in due course, to very useful assistance from the parents.

The Medical Officer of Health now receives information from school visitors, inspectors, teachers, parents and others, of diseases not included under the Notification Act, printed post cards for the purpose being supplied to those responsible; children coming from homes in which *any* inmate is suffering from infectious sickness are excluded from the schools.

Hardship is minimised by a careful application of the powers to exclude individual scholars, because unless this is attended to it is quite possible that disease may rapidly spread to an extent which would render it necessary to close the department or the school altogether, a procedure detrimental to educational interests.

An observation made over a series of years of the number of cases of measles occurring during the three weeks preceding the school holidays, with the number occurring during the three weeks succeeding the holidays, when precisely the same means of notification are in operation, showed that the cases before the holidays outnumbered those after the holidays by about 3 to 1.

The nature of the disease, its character, the number of pupils affected, have been factors in determining the necessity for school closure.

In this connection the value of the records[1] of the infectious illness from which each child has suffered is obvious. If, for example, a child suffering from measles is found in the Infants Department of a school the probable consequences will be less serious and procedure less stringent if the records show that a large proportion of the infants in this class have already suffered from that disease; if none of them have, apprehension will be greater.[2]

[1] Already referred to on p. 120.
[2] See diagram, p. 114.

What applies to public elementary schools, whether designated denominational schools or Council schools, also applies to Sunday schools and private schools; although these latter establishments are not subject to the same supervision by the Sanitary Authority as the others, yet the Public Health Act does make certain provisions which are applicable to schools of every kind, and the managers of these establishments have been perfectly willing to act upon the suggestions which the Sanitary Authority has found necessary to offer.

Financial grants have constituted an important factor in questions of absenteeism and school closure, and the regulations under which grants were made have from time to time been varied; the absence of pupils, unless for valid reasons, resulted in a loss of grant concerning those pupils, but the closure of the entire school, however, did not at all times involve a loss of grant, and consequently there was a considerable period during which a school would suffer less loss of grant if an entire department were closed than if numerous individual scholars were absent. The existence of infectious disease at the home of a pupil was always regarded by the Board of Education, and by the Liverpool Council of Education, as a valid reason for the non-attendance of the children at school, and qualified them to receive any benefits to which regular attendance would have entitled them.

A convalescent child may be free from infection, and therefore, so far as the risk of infection is concerned, may with perfect safety return to school, yet it may not be sufficiently strong to undertake at once the full work and discipline which attendance at school entails; the permission of the Health Department to return to school, therefore, implied nothing further than freedom from infection.

Under the Education Act (1902) the Liverpool City Council becomes the Education Authority, and the important departments of Health and Education are thus enabled to co-operate closely in all matters affecting the health of the scholars. Many thousands of communications relating to this aspect of child welfare pass between the two departments annually.

The appointment of an additional assistant School Medical

Officer of Health was decided upon during the year 1906, partly with a view to noting the physical condition of scholars, but primarily so as to make more efficient the system already in vogue to check the spread from child to child of any communicable infection, including troubles due to neglect and want of cleanliness. The Liverpool Corporation Act of 1908 required parents of school children to notify the Medical Officer of Health and the head teacher of the occurrence of infectious disease in the house within 24 hours of becoming aware of it, and to keep from school the affected children, and any others the Medical Officer of Health considered necessary; the scope of the clause included Sunday schools and all other schools. Parliament had recognised the special circumstances of Liverpool on many occasions, *inter alia*, in allowing a special clause in the Act of 1902, which imposed a penalty of £5 upon any person proved to have given a false answer in reply to inquiries addressed by the Health Authorities as to the existence of infectious disease in the home.

Employment of Children Acts

The Employment of Children Act came into force on January 1, 1904. The Act was designed to prevent the overworking of children under fourteen years of age in those occupations which were then unregulated by law. It was manifest that the employment of young school children until late hours at night could not be other than injurious, and in the extreme cases in which the earnings of the child were looked to for the maintenance of its parents, relief through the established channels was preferable to risk to the child's health. The Act empowered the Council to make byelaws prescribing the conditions and hours of employment; to regulate street trading by persons under the age of sixteen years, to determine the days and hours during which, and the places at which, such street trading may be carried on, and the conditions of the employment of children in barbers' shops.

The Education Act of 1918, and the byelaws made thereunder (which, however, did not come into operation until April 1, 1920), further restricted the employment of children liable to attend school; the age of twelve was substituted for eleven years, and the total hours of employment on school days were reduced from three and a half to two hours—no child being permitted to commence work before 7 a.m. or be employed after 7 p.m. On Saturdays or school holidays, the period of employment was reduced, and on Sundays, no child could be employed in any occupation other than as a chorister or in the delivery of milk, and the employment was confined to two hours between 8 a.m. and 10 a.m.

No child could be employed before school hours (and then only for one hour) unless he or she received a certificate signed by the School Medical Officer that the employment would not be prejudicial to the child's health nor render the child unfit to obtain the proper benefit from its education.

It is interesting to observe that on April 30, 1915, when the byelaws under the Employment of Children Act, 1903, were in operation, the number of "employed" school children in Liverpool was 3082; this number was reduced to 1698 in 1921, while at the end of 1926 the corresponding figure was 1522. At the end of 1929 the number on the register was 1627.

So far as street trading is concerned no girl under sixteen years of age may be employed, and only boys over fourteen who have been licensed.

Care of Defective Children

In 1893, under the Blind and Deaf Children Act, the School Boards had accepted the responsibility of providing for the education of the blind and the deaf. It is well known that a large proportion of the cases of blindness were preventable; nearly 40 per cent. of all cases of blindness in children were due to ophthalmia which newly born infants acquired at birth from an ailment affecting the mother. In 1909 a small ward of four beds, later increased to ten, was provided at St Paul's Eye Hospital,[1] and at all times the midwives gave valuable co-operation to the scheme.[2]

As early as June, 1899, thus anticipating Parliamentary action by many years, the Liverpool School Board decided to make special provision for the education of both mentally and physically defective children, and special schools were provided for

[1] See p. 110.   [2] See p. 113.

this purpose, the first being opened at Shaw Street in 1900. Four other special schools were opened within the next four years and a special part-time Medical Officer appointed by the Education Committee for supervising the children admitted to these schools.

In 1909 the Education Committee obtained permission from the Council to alter and equip Bowring House, a mansion situated on an estate at Roby—which had been given to the city by the late Sir William Bowring—temporarily as a residential school for the children belonging to the schools for the physically defective; in 1924 this school was discontinued, alternative premises with accommodation for sixty children of both sexes having been secured at Woolton Vale.

Provision of Meals for Necessitous School Children

About thirty years ago a system of feeding necessitous school children was inaugurated by certain teachers and other philan-thropists, the funds being provided by voluntary subscription; the system was subsequently developed by the Education Com-mittee. Coupons were issued to schools which desired them, and were made available at the British Workman Cocoa Rooms. A committee, known as the Underfed Children's Meals Com-mittee, working in close co-operation with the Education Committee, was formed, and centres were opened in some of the elementary schools, mission halls, etc.

This system, which was in full operation when the Education (Provision of Meals) Act, 1906, came into force, continued until 1910, when a sub-committee of the Education Committee was established to put the Act into operation, and to arrange for the feeding of the necessitous children under the committee's direct control. In 1915 arrangements were made for the meals to be cooked at the several day industrial schools, upon an approved dietary drawn up by the Medical Officer of Health.

No charge is made for the meals, but only such children are eligible whose parents' income comes within a scale laid down by the committee.

Medical Inspection of School Children

The Education Act of 1902 had involved the taking over of all the public elementary schools, including voluntary schools, by the City Council, which had been constituted the Local Education Authority. All existing school buildings were inspected and reported upon by the Director of Education, the Surveyor, and the Medical Officer of Health; a number of the older schools were closed as unsuitable, and more or less extensive structural alterations were made in others.

This work was still in progress when in 1908 the Board of Education initiated the highly important work of medical inspection of school children, the aims being to determine the physical condition of the children, their fitness to benefit from the educational opportunities afforded in the public elementary schools, the early detection of commencing disease, the sufficiency or otherwise of feeding and other matters affecting their physical welfare. The views formulated by the Board of Education were inserted in the Education (Administrative Provisions) Act of 1907, and the City Council was given:

The duty to provide for the medical inspection of children immediately before or at the time of, or as soon as possible after, their admission to a public elementary school, and on such other occasions as the Board of Education direct, and the power to make such arrangements as may be sanctioned by the Board of Education for attending to the health and physical welfare of the children.

Parliament, recognising the valuable work already done by progressive local authorities, aided by generous voluntary effort, "provided that in any exercise of powers under the section the Local Education Authority may encourage and assist the establishment or continuance of voluntary agencies and associate with itself representatives of voluntary agencies and voluntary associations for the purpose".

Controversy arose at the outset, as to how the medical inspection should be conducted; the Education Committee, to whom the City Council referred the matter, was disposed to act upon the view that an entirely new medical organisation was necessary, wholly divorced from the general public health administration of the city, and that the Medical Officers should confine their duties solely to the examination of the children, and act under the instructions of the director of elementary education. This view, however, was not shared by the Board of Education nor by the City Council which, having regard to the closeness of the association which already existed between the school children and the Medical Officer of Health and his staff, decided that the work should be carried out in conjunction with the existing Medical Department. Three assistant School Medical Officers were appointed to give their whole time to this important work, and the part-time services of seven other medical men, who had already been investigating the subject of the insufficient or improper feeding of school children, were temporarily retained.

A circular letter was sent to the head teacher of each department explaining the objects of the inspection and the inspecting Medical Officer called upon the head teachers a few days before the inspection of the school to arrange the work with a minimum of interference with school duties; the sympathy and co-operation of the school teachers were readily secured. The Board of Education provided a form in which a record of the results of the examination might conveniently be kept; parents were invited to attend the examination—which at that time they seldom did—and, if present, were informed of the nature of defects found, and if necessary were advised to consult their doctor without delay. When the parents did not attend, a notice was sent to them explaining any defect found.

The Queen Victoria District Nursing Association had by arrangement with the Education Committee already provided for the attendance of nurses in thirty-eight schools to deal with minor injuries and with conditions arising from lack of cleanliness. In order to help the newly appointed medical inspectors the Health Committee placed the services of some of the health visitors at their disposal to assist with the children, and in recording their height, weight, condition as to cleanliness, etcetera, and to "follow up" the children and to ascertain that instructions were given effect to.

At the outset it was found to be not an unusual thing for

children in the lower parts of the city to wear the same number of garments summer and winter, and not infrequently their clothes were stitched on and unchanged probably for weeks or months, a condition to which Dr Arkle, who had given much thought to the welfare of school children, had already drawn attention. The visits of the health visitors to the homes of children found to be verminous enabled the Health Department to deal with them under the Liverpool Corporation Act of 1908, into which a clause had been introduced to meet this evil, whilst another very important general Act, the Children Act of 1908, also gave powerful support in the same direction. The Health Committee authorised its staff to convey children who were found to be verminous to the Charters Street Disinfecting Station, where special washing accommodation and facilities for disinfection of clothing were available; later the Baths Committee sanctioned the use of a cleansing station for a certain number of children at Mansfield Street Baths; the cost was almost wholly provided by the Health Committee, whose staff, notably the female staff, rendered most valuable assistance.

Numbers of children of the poorest class and below school age, with whom the Education Committee had no concern but who required attention in this connection, had been cared for by the Health Committee, an arrangement which pointed the way for that body ultimately taking over the whole responsibility. At the outset the provision for cleansing was far from meeting the necessities of the case, and, in due course, special cleansing stations were provided which met the needs of a happily diminishing evil.

Medical inspection revealed the effects upon school life of the so-called industrial employment of children, a subject already referred to. The evil of insufficient sleep, usually resulting from young children being allowed by their parents to play in the street till late at night, was also brought into notice.

For the treatment of the varied ailments the general and special hospitals and dispensaries, and the Dental Hospital, were the only available places for treatment at the initiation of the work, but the large number of children requiring attention for minor ailments overwhelmed these establishments and imposed calls upon them to which the staffs were unable to respond, and the necessity for special school clinics was early foreshadowed.

As the work progressed experience showed that the decision to co-ordinate as intimately as possible the work of the medical inspection of school children with that of the Public Health Department was very fully justified by the results.

The presence at the inspections of members of the female staff of the Public Health Department enabled them to ascertain which were the homes especially needing supervision, and in this way not only the particular child but the whole household benefited, the school proving the short cut to the dirty homes.

Objections to the inspection on the part of the parents were exceedingly few, and were usually due to a misunderstanding of its aim and scope, or in a few cases, apparently, in order that the neglected condition of the child might not be brought to light.

The Police Aided Clothing Association provided clothes for many of the scholars, the female sanitary staff referring parents to this association for assistance.[1]

Tuberculosis received the special attention of the school medical staff, and a number of actual or doubtful cases which were brought to light were attended to by members of the honorary staff of the Liverpool Consumption Hospital.

The Education Committee, under the Education (Administrative Provisions) Act, and later under the Education Act, 1921, made provision for advancing the cost of spectacles when there was great poverty, the parents undertaking, where able, to refund the money in weekly payments. In a few instances the assistance of the Poor Law Authorities was obtained by the parents in this connection.

A great want of consideration was shown by parents respecting care of the teeth, and only the likelihood of proceedings for neglect led to attention to needs. At the Harrington Council School an experimental dental clinic was instituted at the end of 1910 for children attending that school.

By 1913 there were 160 public elementary schools with 130,000 scholars on the rolls, infants below five years of age being no longer admitted to the schools. The examination of

---

[1] See p. 109.

children at the age of twelve instead of at the age of thirteen was recommended, as this would give a reasonable time in which any defects found might be remedied before the children left school. Stammerers classes and defective vision classes were instituted.

Personal hygiene, temperance and physical exercises were taught in all the schools, the syllabus being on the lines of that drawn up by the Board of Education and the teachers supplied with standard text-books on the subjects.

In 1913 a clinic for treatment of ringworm of the scalp by means of X-rays was opened at the North Corporation School in view of the protracted absence from school due to ringworm. To meet visual defects two eye specialists were appointed to attend the clinic, and sixteen practitioners, specially qualified, were appointed to see children at their own consulting rooms at a fee of five shillings per completed case; parents were thus able to select a doctor most convenient for their homes. A financial standard was fixed in order to prevent the children of parents who could afford a private doctor being treated under the committee's scheme.

In 1914, after the outbreak of War, and the departure of most of the staff, available part-time Medical Officers were utilised and the work slowly developed, but the examination of the intermediate group of children at the age of eight had to be relinquished. During the previous year certain of the hospitals had intimated their inability to continue to treat the increasing number of cases of enlarged tonsils and adenoids detected at school medical inspections, the committee therefore at the close of the War, in 1919, decided to open a clinic at the North Dispensary, and twelve beds were provided in a dormitory to allow of the children operated on staying the night. A charge varying from 2*s*. 6*d*. to 10*s*. was made, according to the parents' income. This clinic at once proved to be very popular. Another had been opened in Old Swan during 1917 for the treatment of cases of defective vision, and various clinics for the treatment of minor ailments were opened in suitable districts.[1]

An exhaustive inquiry was carried out in 1920 into the frequency, causation, treatment, etcetera, of crippling in children of school

[1] See Annual Reports to the Education Committee by the School Medical Officer.

age. This inquiry gave, for the first time, an estimate of the prevalence of crippling and an idea of the problems awaiting solution It showed that in almost 36 per cent. of the cases the crippling was the result of surgical tuberculosis; in nearly 24 per cent. it was due to paralysis; in over 15 per cent. to rickets, and in nearly 14 per cent. of the cases it was due to heart disease.

It was further ascertained that in 60 per cent. of the cases the defects had existed before the age of five, that is to say, before school life. The desirability of establishing better arrangements for earlier detection and treatment of the cases of crippling led to closer co-operation between the various agencies interested. During 1921 an Aural Clinic was added to the Minor Ailments Clinic.

A short summary for a single year (1929) will give an idea of the nature and the extent of the comprehensive functions of the school medical service. In the elementary schools the number of inspections of children in 1929 amounted to 102,227, the number of inspections of pupils attending the higher schools was 13,247. A thorough examination of each school and a full report on the conditions of the school premises are made annually. Children absent from school for various defects are examined periodically at special centres; these examinations in 1929 numbered 4222. In every case where defects are found notices are sent to parents with information as to how the necessary treatment may be obtained, and school nurses who have been specially trained for the work attend at the examinations and at the clinics. The number of children and the defects treated are shown in the following table:

Defects treated	No. of clinics	No. of children treated during 1929
Minor ailments	7	13,160
Defective vision	3	5,846
Ringworm of the scalp	1	209
Dental defects	4	15,570
Tonsils and adenoids	1	1,363
Aural defects	2	701
Scabies	2	249

Special Schools. The Certifying Officers examined over 1000 children with regard to their suitability for attendance at the day or residential schools for the mentally and physically defective. The Medical Officers also conducted over 2000 examinations of the children in attendance at these schools.

Although the activities of the school medical service have more than realised the anticipations of those who first urged the necessity for such a service, its full development has not yet been reached.

Whilst the arrangements for the detection of defects can be regarded as fairly complete, there is much more that will eventually be done in the direction of prevention and treatment; in Liverpool there are at present several important out-patient orthopaedic departments attached to hospitals, and a very valuable voluntary agency, the Child Welfare Association, helping in this matter.

With regard to the prevalence of rheumatism and frequency of serious effects on the heart, more might be done to limit or prevent such complications in further provision of special hospital accommodation and also residential school accommodation where the cases can be kept under careful supervision after discharge from hospital. For delicate children in whom the defect is not so pronounced as to necessitate residential treatment, open-air day schools within reasonable access of their homes are desirable. No special provision has been made for the early detection and treatment of mental ailments; it is a matter for consideration whether a special clinic to which neuropathic or unstable children could be referred for investigation would be advantageous.

On consideration of the records of the medical examinations of school children, one is struck by the large number of entrants who are found with various untreated defects; the most frequent defects found being dental caries, defective eyesight, chest troubles, diseases of the ear, nose and throat, and deformities.

The Health Authority deals with the child from birth to the age of five, the most critical and important age from the health standpoint; efforts however have been mainly concentrated upon the infant during the first twelve months of age, with results which have been almost phenomenal in their success,[1] and to a considerable extent the second year of life has been similarly safeguarded. Between three and five, however, the supervision is not so close and might be extended with advantage.

[1] See p. 108.

Chapter VII

WATER SUPPLY

Early provision—Scarcity, high price and theft of water—Disputes and appeals to Magistrates—Wells—Rivington—Uses of salt water —Growing demands—Further sources of supply—Hawes-water or Vyrnwy—Chemical and bacteriological examinations—Vyrnwy and afforestation schemes—Compulsory limit of supply—Drought and waste from frost—Pipe lines and extensions of distributing mains—Acts of Parliament concerned—Baths and Wash-houses— Early provision—Extensions—Importance as health accessories.

THE earlier sources of water supply in Liverpool were shallow wells scooped out of the New Red Sandstone, the principal well in or near Liverpool being situated at the south end of the land now occupied by St George's Hall. Prior to 1786 water carts were employed in the distribution of water at the rate of one halfpenny per bucketful, the carts being described as "dangerous vehicles, encumbering the streets, often stopping the narrow ones entirely, or unexpectedly crossing the way of passengers, as they seldom proceed but in a zigzag direction". In 1786 a Local Act of Parliament was obtained to enable the Corporation to contract with owners of land for the supplies of water.

In 1799 a private Act incorporated a company entitled "The Company of Proprietors of the Liverpool Waterworks" for "better supplying the Town and Port of Liverpool with water from certain streams in the Parish of Bootle". Wooden mains eight inches in diameter, made by hollowing out tree trunks, were constructed by the company, a number of which are now in the Museum of the University School of Hygiene.

In 1822 a private Act incorporated a second private company. This took over such powers as the Corporation had in its 1786 Act. "Thus two rival Companies came into existence and entered into competition for customers. During the first years of their existence they laid pipes side by side in the same streets, and tried to win customers by the usual devices of rival trades-men. But they soon discovered that this competition would be ruinous to both, and they agreed to divide the area of supply, so that, within defined limits, each Company should have a monopoly and be free to make any charge that the Acts of Parliament would permit."[1]

The *Report of the Health of Towns Commission*, 1844, describes their position:

The water which is supplied by the Companies is extremely pure and good.... In the poorer neighbourhoods there is usually a cock in each court, and the inhabitants carry the water and store it in jugs or wooden vessels from day to day; but compared with the dense population, the supply is totally inadequate, as the turncocks of the Company cannot allow it to run a sufficient length of time, and many of the poorer inhabitants (whether from this circumstance, or from inherent habits of filth, I do not venture to say) have never had their boarded floors properly scoured since the houses were erected. Many of the poor beg water, many steal it, and if the Companies were to prosecute all such cases, I apprehend that the magistrates would not find time for much other employment. The complaints as to the scarcity of water in cases of fire, and also as to the present prices of the much needed commodity, are both loud and general, but the Companies, who have a valuable property in the monopoly, and whose shares are at such a high premium, do not see fit to lower their prices; and so long as both Companies have a mutual understanding they may advance the price, or make specific agreements as favourable to themselves as they choose.

The danger to the prosperity of the town from the deficient supply became so serious that the matter was at length taken in hand by the Highway Commissioners, and in 1843 they promoted a Bill to provide for an independent supply for watering the streets, cleansing the sewers, and for extinguishing fires.

The Committee of the House of Commons found the preamble proved, but passed the following resolutions:

1st. That it is the opinion of the Committee that it is essential that an additional supply of water should be afforded to the town of Liverpool, to be applied to the extinguishing of fires and certain other public purposes, and to be kept distinct from the supply for domestic purposes.

2nd. That evils are incident to the employment of salt water

[1] Memo. prepared by Mr Joseph Parry, Water Engineer, in 1903 for the *Handbook of the Liverpool Congress of the Royal Institute of Public Health.*

generally and exclusively to the extinguishing of fires, which it appears to the Committee desirable, if possible, to avoid incurring.

3rd. That an additional supply of fresh water, available and sufficient for the prompt and effectual extinction of fires, can be best afforded by laying a new system of mains, and larger in dimensions than those generally used by the Harrington Company, which (new) mains shall be kept continually charged.

Thus, a Bill promoted for the purpose of enabling the Commissioners to supply the town with salt water became, by the action of Parliament, an Act for a new supply of fresh water, and resulted in the sinking of the famous Green Lane Well.

It is an interesting side-light that at this period the magistrates complained that most of their time was taken up in settling brawls and strife among the inhabitants of the lower class of the city which arose in the competition for water.

The Report of the Commissioners who conducted the preliminary Parliamentary inquiry with respect to the Bill of 1847 shows the state of things which prevailed under the Companies:

In some cases the water is not supplied for a longer time than for a quarter of an hour to half an hour, and that only on alternate days; that the water is sometimes laid on as late as eleven o'clock at night, and as early as six o'clock in the morning; that the supply is not sufficient for domestic purposes; and that frequent complaints are made as to the uncertainty of water coming in; that in numerous instances the supply is by a standpipe or tap, from which the inhabitants of the courts have to be supplied during the time the water is on; they are therefore obliged to store what they can thus obtain in jars and casks; that in many cases they have to beg for water, and in others to borrow it; the want of water causes people to use it over and over again.

Having adopted the Rivington scheme, on the advice of Mr Hawkesley, for impounding the upper waters of the Rivers Douglas and Roddlesworth in Lancashire, the Corporation obtained the Liverpool Water Works Act of 1848 authorising the construction of the Rivington works; when the Act was before a committee of the House of Lords it was opposed by Rivington landowners, and clauses designed to prevent the fouling of the water, which had been inserted by Parliament in the general Water Works Clauses Act earlier in the same year, were struck out of the Bill and thus Liverpool was deprived by the House of Lords of the protection which under the general law applied to all waterworks undertakings. In 1871 the Corporation made successful application to Parliament to restore the clauses which had been rejected twenty-three years previously.

The Rivington scheme was denounced by a large body of voters and others outside the Council as an unnecessary expense, and Mr W. Rathbone, the Chairman, who had advocated the scheme, consequently lost his seat for the ward which he represented; other supporters may have shared that fate, being regarded as delegates, expected to vote as directed, and not upon information placed before them—to know what is good and do what is bad.

In 1849 the questions at issue were referred by the Council to Mr Robert Stevenson, who in 1850 reported in favour of the Rivington works. These were commenced in 1852, and the water first delivered in Liverpool in 1857, additions to the local supplies meanwhile being made by the sinking of wells to meet the growing demands.

The Act of 1847 contemplated, and indeed required, the Corporation to give a constant supply, a requirement that was modified in the Liverpool Water Works Act, 1862, which enacted "that the water to be supplied by the Corporation under the Waterworks Act and this Act respectively, need not be laid on under a pressure or supplied to an elevation greater than can be afforded by gravitation from their works".

When the Rivington water was first brought to Liverpool the filter beds were not wholly efficient, and the water had a brownish tinge which dissatisfied the people. Consequently the supply of well-waters was continued from such wells as attained a sufficient standard of purity, but all the wells, with the exception of Windsor, formerly belonging to the company, were abandoned.

The demand for water rapidly increased as the town grew; additional powers were sought at the Parliamentary Session, 1866, to purchase water discharged into the Roddlesworth, to construct a new reservoir at Rivington, and also to sink two new wells, one at Dudlow Lane, and the other at Bootle.

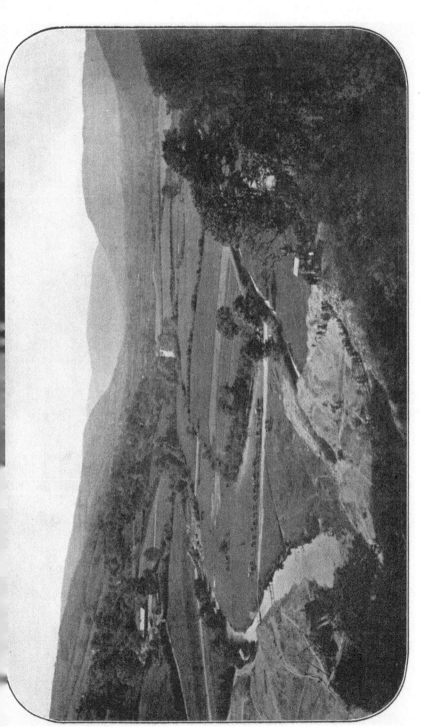

The Vyrnwy Valley prior to the construction of the masonry dam.

In 1873, and for several succeeding years, the Council had under consideration the importance of obtaining supplies from really adequate sources; Bala Lake, Derwent-water, Lake Windermere, Hawes-water, and the River Vyrnwy, were all carefully considered, and the consulting engineers, Hawkesley and Deacon, concluded that Vyrnwy possessed all the more important advantages of Hawes-water, with some indeed which the latter did not possess. Both waters are soft, and very pure. It is interesting to note that the Manchester Council is now adopting Hawes-water as an additional supply for that city. Vyrnwy being finally decided upon, the impounding of the river was commenced in 1888. In July 1891, water was first sent through the Vyrnwy Aqueduct to Liverpool, and the works were formally opened in July 1892. The original pipe line was supplemented by a second in 1904.

In 1887, when the Vyrnwy works were approaching completion, drought greatly imperilled the supply to the city; among other methods of temporary relief special mains were laid from the Pier Head in order to distribute salt water to the swimming baths, for watering streets in the centre of the city, and for flushing drains and sewers.

The results of chemical and bacteriological examinations of water stored in domestic cisterns evidenced the advantage of a direct supply from the mains for drinking purposes and the need for further Parliamentary powers to minimise pollution at Rivington; the increasing population of surrounding districts made it clear that purchase of the watershed afforded the only means of effective protection. The Liverpool Corporation Act of 1902 empowered the Corporation to purchase practically the whole of the Rivington gathering-ground, with the exception of Lever Park, a gift made by the late Lord Leverhulme to his native town of Bolton, and which was adequately safeguarded. The Corporation already had 4000 acres, leaving 5000 acres, which were acquired under the compulsory clauses of the Act.

In 1903 the planting of the Vyrnwy watershed was under consideration with the advice of Professor Fisher of the Forestry Department, Royal Engineering College, and extensive schemes of afforestation were promoted.

The year 1904 was characterised by long continuance of hot dry weather and unusually heavy demands upon the water resources.

The completion in the following year of the second line of supply enabled the demands of the steadily increasing population to be met. The Vyrnwy scheme was designed to provide for Liverpool a total supply of 40,000,000 gallons of sand-filtered water daily; the total quantities of water supplied during 1905 from each of the respective sources, but omitting the salt water, were Vyrnwy 44 per cent., Rivington 43 per cent., wells 13 per cent.

Between the first delivery of Vyrnwy water to Liverpool and the delivery of the second instalment there was an interval of fourteen years. It was thought that a much longer period would elapse before a third instalment would be required.

In 1903 negotiations commenced with Birkenhead as to the best method of obtaining a permanent supply for Birkenhead; to give a *permanent* supply from Lake Vyrnwy necessarily involved an application to Parliament. This was not proceeded with and the negotiations did not materialise.

Compulsory limits of supply are those places where the Corporation has a monopoly of the supply, and where it is bound under statutory obligations to extend its mains and to distribute water. These in 1907 included a total area of 117 square miles, in addition to Chorley, comprising the city of Liverpool and the various adjacent townships which are virtually its outgrowths.

The death of Professor Campbell Brown, who since 1869 had been the Chemical Analyst to the Water Committee, occurred in 1910. He had ably guided that committee on highly important chemical questions during this long period. He was followed as Chemical Analyst by Dr Collingwood Williams, the County Analyst, but his growing duties as County Analyst led him to relinquish the post to his successor Professor W. H. Roberts.

In the following year, 1911, the death occurred of the Bacteriological Analyst, Sir Rubert Boyce; his systematic bacteriological examinations had since 1900 included a daily examination

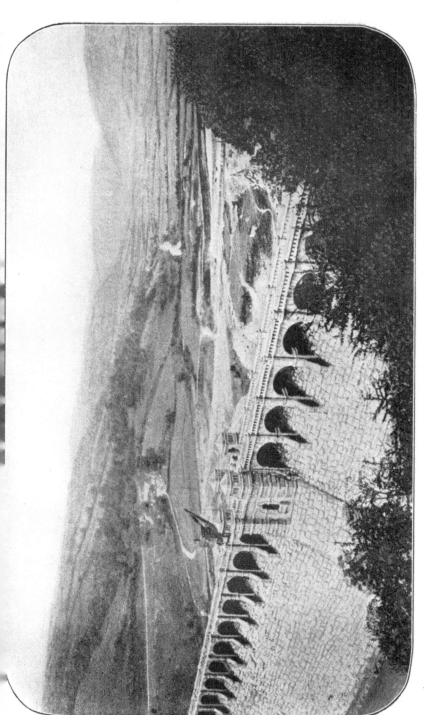

The completed dam and the submergence of the Valley.

of the water delivered from various mains in the city, a procedure which has been continued.

Upon the death of Sir Rubert Boyce, Professor Ernest Glynn temporarily undertook duty pending the appointment of Professor Beattie in 1912.[1]

The year 1914 marked the retirement of Mr Joseph Parry, who for many years filled the important and responsible office of Water Engineer; his successor, Colonel Davidson, left for service in France, and Mr Parry resumed the office during the War, a period which suspended all new works, excepting such as were absolutely necessary; supplies of water were afforded to the large military camps in the neighbourhood of the city, as well as to the various military hospitals, defence enclosures, munition works, etcetera.

In 1917, two circumstances happened to tax the resources of waterworks with exceptional severity, one a spell of intense frost, the other a long summer drought. Of the two, frost exacts the greater strain owing to the great waste from burst pipes which cannot be easily or quickly dealt with. From a sanitary point of view, however, the demand during a hot dry summer is a more serious matter.[2]

In 1919 the total supply of water to the city reached 15,604,000,000 gallons, and it is interesting to note that of this Vyrnwy now contributed 65·1 per cent., Rivington 28·7 per cent., and the wells 6·2 per cent. Vyrnwy had furnished 350,000,000 gallons more than in the preceding year. A national shortage of fuel had imposed a new limitation to the quantity of water raised from the wells, and the added supply from Vyrnwy facilitated an economy in coal for pumping.

Nearly two miles of new distributing mains were laid during the year 1920 in the city and suburbs, although the work was interfered with by trade disputes.

The Liverpool Corporation Water Works Act of 1920 facilitated in certain particulars the construction of the third pipe line from Vyrnwy to take advantage of the fact, already alluded to, that the Vyrnwy watershed yielded a greater supply

[1] See p. 190.
[2] See pp. 76, 179.

than was estimated in 1880. A fourth pipe line was also contemplated under the 1920 Act.

In 1925 the average daily quantity sent out from the works for all purposes, excepting compensation water to rivers, was approximately 41,823,000 gallons, and the amount supplied to the city and suburbs per day per head of population was represented by 34·6 gallons.[1]

The growing city necessitated considerable increase in new distributing mains, the Corporation housing schemes being responsible for very considerable lengths.[2]

The use of the new trunk main from Prescot enabled a greatly improved pressure to be maintained in several districts where it was formerly deficient, but the developments of new housing extensions and other claims were rendering it imperative to take immediate steps to bring additional water into Liverpool from Vyrnwy, notwithstanding that the existing mains, as well as the Rivington aqueduct, were taxed to their utmost capacity and the wells were being drawn upon to an increased extent. The scheme had been authorised by the City Council in 1919, but the inauguration was postponed owing to the excessive cost of work at that period. During the year 1926 the Water Committee decided to proceed with the work of the third pipe line.

During the year 1927 the diminution in industrial activities consequent upon the coal dispute diminished the demand for water by 1,500,000 gallons daily as compared with the previous twelve months. The coal dispute also delayed for several months the procedure with the third pipe line, but by the middle of February 1927, considerable progress had been made.

The districts within the compulsory area of supply included the city of Liverpool and Bootle, and the districts of Eccleston, Hale, Halewood, Knowsley, Speke, Tarbock, Whiston, Rainhill, Prescot, Great Crosby, Little Crosby, Litherland, Waterloo with Seaforth, Ford, Aintree, Croxteth Park, Huyton, Ince Blundell, Kirkby, Lunt, Netherton, Sefton, Simonswood, Thornton and West Derby. The estimated population of the area

[1] See Annual Reports of Water Engineer.
[2] See Housing Operations.

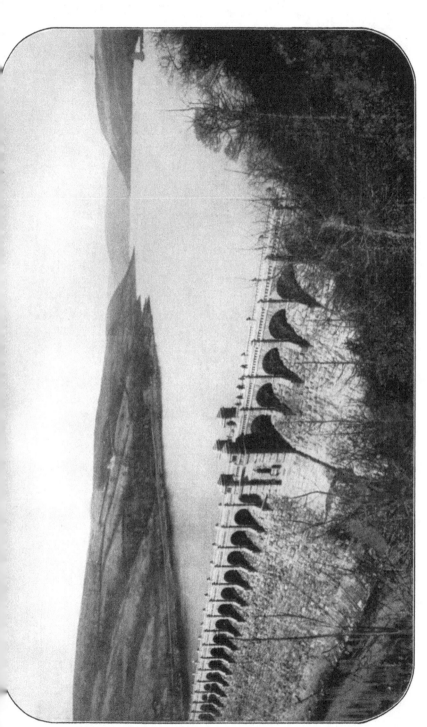

View of masonry dam across the Vyrnwy Valley, and the conversion of the Valley into the Lake.

within the limits of compulsory supply based on the 1921 census was 1,027,227, apart from the districts supplied by agreement. The total quantity of water supplied during the year ending March 31, 1927, inside and outside the compulsory limits of supply, was 15,584,533,000 gallons; the gallon is an inconvenient unit, its translation into tons would give a figure more appreciable. The amount of compensation water, that is, water supplied from Lake Vyrnwy to obviate the possibility of loss to districts lower down the river, is 10,000,000 gallons per day, and is more than five times the dry weather flow of the rivers; these districts derive the additional advantages of uniformity as well as purity of supply. The supply to Liverpool is 35 gallons per head per day, all the water being filtered. There is a constant supply of a perfectly pure, filtered water, delivered at any floor of every house, transported sixty-eight miles from the hills of Wales, for the small cost of $1\frac{1}{2}d.$ a ton. The purity of the watersheds is carefully protected under Parliamentary powers, and there is a system of inspection by wharfsmen and reservoir men to ensure protection of the areas from pollution, whilst analysis, both chemical and bacteriological, of the water as delivered in Liverpool is made, and the testing and stamping of water fittings constitute an important part of the work of the Water Department.

Thirty-seven Acts of Parliament are concerned with the Liverpool water supply, the earliest dating from the reign of Queen Anne, when in 1709 Parliament authorised the construction of works to convey water to Liverpool from wells in Bootle. Many of these Acts having served their purpose were repealed, the remainder have been consolidated in Part IV of the Consolidation Act of 1921, a sarcophagus in which their dates and the circumstances which occasioned their needs and the historic interest associated with them lie interred.

Baths and Wash-houses

The community bath founded in 1789 by the Jewish population in connection with the Frederick Street Synagogue was the first bath founded in Liverpool. At the beginning of last century

there were no public baths in Liverpool; a private bathing
establishment, started some years afterwards, was situated close
to and gave its name to Bath Street. The Corporation purchased
this private establishment for £40,000 and made large alterations.
"By this expenditure", says an anonymous local historian, "the
baths have all the advantages of the salubrity of salt water
without exposing the bather to public view." On the construction of the Princes Dock in 1822 the Corporation proceeded
with the baths at St George's Pier, notwithstanding that a
memorial addressed to "our public and spirited chief magistrate,
and signed by 130 of the most respectable parties in Liverpool,
was presented against it", on the grounds mainly that it would
not meet the needs of invalids and females. These baths were
managed by the Council up till 1836, when they were let to a
Mrs Penn.

Meanwhile, in 1832, when cholera ravaged the town, the
necessity of cleanliness as a means of arresting the disease
became apparent. Families, healthy and sick, huddled together
in a single apartment, often an underground cellar, had no means
of helping themselves.

It was left for one of their own class and station, Mrs Catherine
Wilkinson, of Frederick Street, to provide a remedy. She, the wife
of a labourer, living in one of the worst and most crowded streets of
the town, allowed her poorer neighbours, destitute of the means of
heating water, to wash their clothes in the back kitchen of her humble
abode, and to dry them in the covered passage and back yard belonging
to it. Aided by the District Provident Society, and some benevolent
ladies, this courageous self-denying woman contrived to provide for
the washing of, on an average, 85 families per week.

This, begun during the visitation of the cholera, she continued for
several years; the poor people contributing 1d. per week to assist in
defraying the expenses. The supporters of Mrs Wilkinson in her
praiseworthy efforts were Mr and Mrs W. Rathbone and other
beneficent friends.

Stimulated by the success of the scheme, a site was obtained
by the Council in Upper Frederick Street, and building on a
very humble scale was proceeded with as an experiment. In
May 1841, the first public establishment of baths and wash-
houses for washing clothes in this country was opened. They

were too small and too confined to meet the needs of those who attended, and were enlarged at an early date.[1]

This interesting sanitary experiment was extended in 1844, in which year Mr Tinne, the Chairman of the Baths Sub-Committee, supplied information concerning it to Lord Ashley's Society for the Improvement of the Condition of the Working Classes, which desired to establish similar institutions in London. A further establishment was provided in Paul Street in 1846 and unsuccessful proposals were made to erect further baths and wash-houses in other localities. After lengthened deliberation sites were secured in Mould Street at the north end of the town, in Spencer Street, Everton, at the junction of Parliament Street and Smithdown Lane, in High Park Street, and in Cornwallis Street at the southern part of Liverpool. Designs were submitted by Mr Newlands in 1849 for the Cornwallis Street site, and the baths were opened in 1851, the views of the committee then being that the "conjunction of wash-houses with these baths was not desirable".

Meanwhile, the Pier Head Baths remained in the possession of Mrs Penn until 1850. The high charges of these baths limited their use to those who could afford the charges made, and the annual cost of up-keep devolving upon the Town Council was large.

It is not necessary to pursue further the series of extensions and improvements which took place in regard to baths and wash-houses. The sequence of opening, however, was Cornwallis Street Baths, 1851; Margaret Street, 1863; Steble Street, 1872; Westminster Road, 1877; Lodge Lane, 1878; Burrough Gardens, 1879. In 1894 a further step was taken by the Baths Committee in providing open-air baths for the poorest children, attention being frequently drawn to the fact that children were bathing in the polluted water of the canal, a procedure which not infrequently led to disastrous results by drowning. In 1895 the first open-air bath for children was opened at Burlington Street, in close proximity to the canal with which it had to compete. Its success was very marked, and three additional establishments were opened, in Gore Street in 1898, and in

---

[1] *Report on Baths and Wash-houses*, by J. Newlands, 1857, p. 52, Plate 1.

Green Lane and Mansfield Street in 1899. In each of these a cleansing bath was provided in which the children could wash prior to entering the swimming bath. The addition of a covered gymnasium for the use of the children was speedily made.

Washing baths, i.e. a bathing establishment for cleansing purposes only, and without facilities for swimming, were found to be in demand, and the first people's bath of this character was erected in 1902; no bath of this kind had been previously erected anywhere. Further baths were erected in Lister Drive and in Wavertree. The baths, generally speaking, were used by every section of the community, the public wash-houses for washing clothes being used mainly by the poorer classes, and the "professional" washer, i.e. the person who washes for others, made large use of these premises. Further provision has been made in recent years to meet the growing needs of the population.

Public baths and wash-houses are now available in all parts of the city and constitute a very important part of its sanitary adjuncts. It is quite true that of recent years houses are seldom constructed without a bathroom, and in every house erected by the Housing Committee such provision, together with facilities for hot water supply, are made, but, notwithstanding that, the great extent to which the advantages offered by the public baths and wash-houses are taken advantage of is a sufficient evidence of their value.

Chapter VIII

SUPERVISION OF DWELLINGS

*Common Lodging-Houses—Local legislation—Supervision trans-
ferred from police to sanitary officers—Special provision for emigrants and for women—Proposed municipal common lodging-house
—Voluntary provision—Sub-let houses—Difficulties of control—
Methods of supervision—Progressive improvement—Stringent byelaws in 1911—Cellar dwellings—Cellar population in excess of other
towns—Absence of cellar dwellings in Birmingham—Special legislation—Supervision—Restrictions of occupation and gradual closure
—Canal Boats—Registration and control—Families occupying
canal boats usually have a home ashore.*

Common Lodging-Houses

THE difficulties arising from the overcrowding of houses
upon the land found a counterpart in the overcrowding
of the houses themselves by their occupants. Efforts
were first directed to the class of house known as a common
lodging-house, that is, a place casually resorted to for a single
night, but it will be seen that the sub-letting of single rooms to
a whole family, or even to members of more than one family,
constituted a much greater evil than existed in the case of the
common lodging-house.

The provision and control of common lodging-houses for
those who need them has long been recognised as a necessity;
wayfarers, casual labourers, persons in search of work, travellers
of the poorer class—like others—have been, and still are, in the
habit of resorting to places where a bed can be obtained for
a single night, virtually the hotels of the poorer classes, the
accommodation varying with the charges made. An inference
of the conditions in earlier times will be drawn from the
descriptions relating to typhus in 1847.[1]

Prior to the Liverpool Act of 1842 there was no law in existence
to put common lodging-houses under any official supervision.
Mr Thomas Fresh, Inspector of Nuisances,[2] relates that lodgers
were domiciled on pallets of filthy straw, lying side by side as

[1] See p. 43.   [2] See p. 37.

thickly as they could be packed, without any distinction as to age or sex. Cleanliness and ventilation were unthought of, and moreover the lodging-houses of the lower order were frequented by thieves and vagabonds of all descriptions, and hence it was that the police were associated with their supervision. The Liverpool Improvement Act of 1842, an Act with high ideals and full of aspirations many of which were impossible of fulfilment, gave power to register "lodging-houses of an inferior description" used for casual lodgers, and to frame byelaws with certain specified sanitary requirements, one of which was a cubic space of 300 feet for each inmate. The Act had at least the good effect of locating the positions and ascertaining the condition of the existing lodging-houses, and although one half of them failed to comply with the requirements deemed necessary to justify registration, nevertheless considerable numbers of these were placed upon the register, since this was the only means by which authority to enter and inspect the premises could be claimed.

Under the Liverpool Act of 1846 the duty of ascertaining the ventilation of these premises was imposed upon the Medical Officer of Health, a duty which he endeavoured to discharge single-handed as he had no staff to assist him, not even a clerk.

About this time there were 450 common lodging-houses on the register, and in 1847 the Council commenced a supervision by the appointment of the inspectors and sergeants of the police force, about seventy-five in number, to make occasional night visits to common lodging-houses, and to lay information in all cases where the number of lodgers was in excess of those allowed. Supervision, therefore, in this way became, and for many years continued to be, a police and not a health matter, the procedure being justified on the grounds of economy, and of the roughness and criminal tendencies of many of the inmates.

The 1846 Act gave no power to refuse application for registration however unfit the applicant or premises might be, but it did authorise a control in the number of lodgers and in this way gave a control, more or less effective, over these places.

That some supervision was necessary is evidenced by the fact that about a third of the keepers were unable to write, and certainly could not be depended upon to carry out the sanitary requirements unless they were closely watched.

It was gradually recognised that the use of the police force in the sanitation of common lodging-houses was not the most effective, partly because it interfered with their ordinary duties and partly because their visits were looked upon by the inmates as due to criminal rather than advisory reasons, which was no doubt often the case; a later application by the Council for fuller Parliamentary powers resulted in the passing of the Liverpool Sanitary Act of 1866, when the duty of supervision of these places was transferred to the Health Committee, and four officers were specially appointed to give their whole time to the visitation of common lodging-houses. It is interesting to note that the four persons appointed were all ex-police officers, and the practice of employing ex-policemen has been continued, so far as circumstances would permit, up to the present time, since their discipline, character, training and physique were found to be the best basis for the subsequent training—inaugurated in 1883—for their new duties; from the time that they ceased to discharge police functions, they were regarded by the people simply as sanitary officers, and their influence greatly increased.

In view of the nature and character of night inspection to detect overcrowding, e.g. counting the people as they lay in bed, it has always been the practice for two officers to go together, with the special sanction of the Medical Officer of Health.

In 1851 and 1853 Common Lodging-House Acts were passed, and in 1869 the Council repealed all their old byelaws and re-enacted many of them in the form prescribed under the 1851 Act, requiring every lodging-house keeper (*a*) to be registered, (*b*) to exhibit in each room of his lodging-house a card showing how many lodgers may occupy the room, (*c*) to observe cleanliness in regard to the rooms, bedding, blankets, and so forth, (*d*) to notify any infection, (*e*) to count two children under ten as one lodger, (*f*) to provide sufficient washing and sanitary accommodation, (*g*) to keep the windows of every sleeping room fully open at prescribed hours, that the day inspectors may see this requirement is complied with, (*h*) to provide for the separation of the sexes.

The general trend has been for the keepers of the smaller and ill-constructed premises to give up the business, or to move into larger premises; this, and the building of new appropriate places, or the adaptation of fair-sized buildings, led to a reduction in the number of common lodging-houses.

As time progressed, regulations were amended in various ways, not the least being the demand for a larger cubic space per lodger. Furthermore, the medical examination of trans-migrants prior to their embarkation, by doctors attached to the various shipping companies, led to a closer regard to health aspects in conducting the business.

With regard to common lodging-houses for women, these resorted to by the poorer classes have been kept under careful supervision, and philanthropy and private enterprise have made good provision for women of the class likely to resort to a common lodging-house, but who for various reasons desire a better accommodation.

In 1907 a large establishment was opened for the reception of women by the Salvation Army in Netherfield Road. The following year a suggestion was made that the Corporation should build a common lodging-house for women, and the subject of municipal common lodging-houses generally received close attention. At that time there were already twenty-eight registered lodging-houses for women, including the accommo-dation provided by the Young Women's Christian Association, the Liverpool Self Help Society for Girls, the Travellers Aid Society and by others, which indeed had never been fully utilised, notwithstanding the great care and pains taken to attract suitable travellers to these homes in preference to the ordinary lodging-houses for women.

On the suggestion of the Medical Officer of Health the Watch Committee authorised the printing of a small card giving the addresses of all the women's lodging-houses to which a chance wayfarer could be safely sent. This card was kept in the posses-sion of every police constable so that he could direct any woman in search of a respectable lodging where to find it; the same information was put in the steerage cabins of the Irish boats.

As time progressed minor gaps in legislation were filled by amendments, and marked improvement resulted in the places coming within the scope of the regulations; some of them, such for example as the Emigration Houses associated with the great shipping companies,[1] the Salvation Army Hostels, the Church Army Houses, and the Bevington Bush Hostel with 672 beds, easily rank, so far as accommodation goes, with many of the minor hotels, and afford every facility for the sanitary needs of their inmates. Night visits to premises of this character are seldom needed, although registration and its sequelae apply.

The Chinese lodging-houses have, as a rule, been well kept and are conspicuously clean, notwithstanding the age of most of the premises.

Under the Merchant Shipping Act of 1883 a special licence was given in the case of seamen's lodging-houses which enabled the licensee to board vessels arriving in the port and seek for lodgers; when this privilege was withdrawn, the applications for the special licence ceased.

The many advantages which would result in common lodging-houses from the provision of a separate day room, in which lodgers could follow their peculiar inclination to cook their own food, were long recognised, and in a number of the better class houses separate day rooms were provided, but it was not until the passing of the Sanitary Act of 1866 that the Health Committee ruled that all registered common lodging-houses should, in due course, have separate day rooms for their lodgers.

In 1929 the actual number of common lodging-houses on the register had been reduced to 136, providing accommodation for 6375 lodgers.

Sub-let Houses

A far-reaching and more difficult subject has been the control of overcrowding in houses the rooms of which were each sub-let to a different family, an evil accentuated when the dwellings themselves were insanitary, as in the case of court houses or

[1] See p. 11.

even cellars. Sub-letting and overcrowding were linked with the poverty associated with the uncertain earnings of unskilled and ill-paid casual labour.[1] Even in the 'seventies the average earnings of the casual unskilled labourer were about 12*s*. a week (although a man in constant work earned 22*s*. a week), and families so placed were content virtually with any accommodation which afforded shelter; mixing of adults of different sexes was common, sometimes unavoidable, frequently due to negligence and indifference, but its nature will be appreciated by the fact that in scores of cases adult sons and daughters slept in the same room, and even in the same bed with their parents, and adults variously related occupied the same rooms and even the same beds. This offence has happily undergone progressive and marked diminution.

The application of the Act of 1846 was an initial step in exercising some guidance over sub-letting, but any beneficial influences which may have been exercised were swept away in the following year by the influx of 300,000 destitute and fever-stricken persons; the consequences of such an invasion, even with the perfected organisation of to-day, may be imagined, the consequences *then* have been dealt with.[2]

Further steps were made by the Nuisances Removal Act of 1855 which dealt with overcrowding as a "nuisance", whilst clauses inserted in the Liverpool Sanitary Act of 1866, relating to the well ordering of sub-let houses, gave opportunities for more effective control; they enabled the overcrowded sections of the town to be divided into eight districts, to each of which an additional inspector was assigned; their duties during the day comprised the registration, inspection and measuring of all houses occupied by members of more than one family, and night visits between the hours of 12 midnight and 2 a.m. were paid by special instructions of the Medical Officer of Health or the Chief Inspector to ill-conducted houses, or where overcrowding was known to be rife, and also, upon complaints, to houses which had not been placed on the register. The inspectors were instructed to act with care and "to regard every person as sober unless the facts to the contrary are very patent".

[1] See p. 56.   [2] See p. 43.

Under the Act, proceedings were taken against the chief tenant who let off the different rooms, and who was held responsible for the conduct of the families occupying them, known as "room keepers"; there was another stumbling-block, inasmuch as the legal adviser of the Justices held that a house must be regarded as a whole, and not considered overcrowded so long as any one room was only partially occupied; it was in fact a question of overcrowding of the house as a whole and not of individual rooms. The procedure was adopted of placing a ticket in each room specifying the number of adults which it might contain, and the registration was an important step in educating the people as to the uses of the various rooms, and in the inculcation of common necessities for decency and health. The sanitary requirements were administered leniently and every effort made to assist the inmates to avoid the offences for which they were punishable.

The miseries to a family living in one room can be readily conceived—the spread of infection, the incident of childbirth, the implication in the Parliamentary power to remove a dead body from a room in which persons live and sleep, are sufficiently suggestive.

Doctors Parkes and Sanderson comment in their Report in 1871 on the great contrast between common lodging-houses, indifferent though they were, and the houses sub-let in lodgings. "The lodging-houses which are under supervision are all ventilated and kept clean, they present a considerable contrast to the sub-let houses." Speaking of the sub-let houses and court houses they remark:

We were not at all prepared for the wretched appearance of the people and the terrible aspect of poverty disclosed.... These conditions were attributed to three circumstances, the irregularity of the labour market, the improvidence and careless habits of the people, and the great intemperance. It is almost impossible, sub-let as most of the rooms in these houses are, for the people in one room to be clean while the others are dirty, they give up the attempt in despair.[1]

The erection of workmen's dwelling-houses meanwhile proceeded and relieved the evil.

[1] See p. 99.

Year by year as the advantages of supervision became more apparent the actual number of sub-let houses placed on the register steadily increased; in 1868 it was 6267, in 1888, 18,967; by 1900 the grosser offences were largely diminished and the Health Committee were advised that new byelaws could be safely applied removing the difficulties of the old, and asking for a larger cubic space and specially recognising the needs of children in this respect. Such byelaws came into operation in 1901 and thirteen inspectors on the public health staff, each of whom held qualifying certificates of sanitary knowledge, were engaged in their administration. In that year 17,863 night visits were paid, resulting in 1351 persons being convicted of various offences; the progress of events, following the more exacting requirements and the closer supervision, continued to show a gradual diminution in the offences; for example in 1904 the number of houses on the register was 22,401, the night visits were 17,886, and the convictions for offences 1146; in 1911 the number of houses was 18,873, with 21,788 night visits and 526 convictions for offences.

In 1911 the byelaws were further strengthened and placed responsibility upon lodgers as well as upon chief tenants in regard to cleanliness, ventilation and so forth. The requirement of an extra cubic space put a different aspect upon the legal offence of overcrowding, as it reduced the number of persons who might occupy a room. Notwithstanding this, however, although the supervision was, if anything, closer, the actual offence was found to diminish in the most satisfactory manner.

Ten years later, in 1921, while it had been possible to reduce the number of houses on the register to 15,332, the night visits, however, had been increased to 24,851, with the gratifying result that only 45 persons were convicted of offences. The figures for last year, 1929, are instructive. The houses on the register total 15,662, the night visits have been reduced to 16,195, and there were no convictions for offences.

The large provision made for housing has been a very important factor in bringing about these good results.

It may be remarked that one of the allegations brought against slum clearances has been that the action of the Insanitary

Property Committee and the Housing Committee, in so far as the removal of slums is concerned, has resulted in the offence of overcrowding in sub-let houses and cellars, an allegation, it will be seen, quite contrary to fact.

Cellar Dwellings

In Liverpool, cellars have been occupied as dwellings for a great number of years; as long ago as 1802 the Corporation consulted Dr Currie and other physicians of the infirmary and dispensaries on the matter. They advised their discontinuance and suggested "a general survey of these subterranean dwellings, and such means adopted for promoting their salubrity as circumstances permit". Unfortunately this advice was not acted upon; forty years later the evil had grown to dimensions far exceeding the occupation of cellars in other towns, the proportion of the working class inhabiting cellars in Liverpool in 1842 being estimated at 20 per cent. against Manchester's 11 per cent.; Birmingham, happily, was wholly free from the trouble.

When the Liverpool Act of 1842 was promoted, no medical opinion was asked for, and a proposal to consult the physicians of the dispensaries was negatived, which may explain shortcomings in that far-reaching Act. The separate occupation of any cellar less than 7 feet in height, or the floor of which was more than 5 *feet below* the level of the street, was prohibited. Under this Act some 3000 of the worst cellars were compulsorily cleared of their inmates, and in the next Act, namely the Liverpool Sanitary Act of 1847, the Council obtained powers to prevent the occupation as a dwelling of any cellar the floor of which was more than 4 *feet below* the ground, and re-affirmed other requirements.

At the time this Act came into operation there were in the borough 7668 cellars used as dwellings housing 30,000 inmates. Of the inhabited cellars 5869 were found on inspection to be damp, wet, or filthy; many were used also for various purposes in addition to that of a dwelling, for example storage of vegetables, fruit, foodstuffs, and other things hawked by the occupants, and, curiously enough, for the slaughtering of animals;

many still had wells of stagnant water sunk in the floor for the purpose of drainage.

Mr Thomas Fresh, who was appointed Inspector of Nuisances under the Act, organised the registration and measurement of the cellars with the aid of four police officers who had been practical tradesmen.

The operations of the Act were attended with great benefit, and led gradually to the closure of cellars and the removal of some thousands of their occupants in succeeding years until under further legislation, new regulations were adopted under the Liverpool Improvement Act of 1871, which prohibited such use of any cellar "the floor of which is more than 4 feet below the level of the street"; the minimum height was required to be 7 feet and in every cellar dwelling a window, water supply and sanitary conveniences were required. Four years later, under the Public Health Act of 1875, somewhat similar requirements were extended to cellar dwellings in all parts of the country.

There was a continued tendency, owing to the influx of families seeking work, to add to the number of cellar dwellings, by letting as separate dwellings cellars which had hitherto only been used in conjunction with the other parts of the house, a practice which re-introduced many objectionable features; in the early 'eighties, cellars illegally occupied, or simply used as deposits for rubbish, were, at the request of the owners, filled in by the Health Committee free of charge; up to the year 1895 about 1000 had been dealt with in this way, but at that date there were still upon the register 9000 cellar dwellings which housed a population of approximately 26,000, the conditions of occupation being however very different from those described as existing in the 'forties.

During the next ten years, with closer supervision, and with the better housing accommodation provided by the Corporation, the number of these unwholesome habitations steadily declined, and in 1905 they were reduced to approximately 3000, housing some 9000 people.

In the following year, 1906, a proposal was put forward to obtain powers under a new Act of Parliament to prevent the occupation of any cellar dwelling after a lapse of four years from the passing of the Act, compensation being paid to the owners, the object of the time-limit being to enable the cellar population to adjust itself under more sanitary conditions. The Health Committee approved of the proposition, which however failed to pass the Council, and the clause was omitted from the Bill; in 1908 the proposal to close and give compensation was again brought forward and this time accepted by the Council, upon the condition that application of the clause should be limited to cellars the floor of which was more than 2 *feet below* the ground; practically all the cellars of the city came within the definition, and the result was the same as it would have been had the suggestions been adopted two years earlier.

The powers granted by Parliament to Liverpool in 1908 were well in advance of anything granted hitherto in respect of cellar dwellings, and it does not appear that these powers have been incorporated in any General Act.

A census taken at the time showed that there were 1793 cellars occupied as dwellings, their total population being 5379. At the expiration of the four years' grace there was a rapid reduction, and in 1914 the number had shrunk to 197, housing a population of 600. Many of the tenants who had formerly occupied cellars were accommodated in the newly erected Corporation houses.

With the War further action was stayed, and owing to the serious shortage of houses at the close of the War there was a tendency to re-occupy cellars as separate dwellings, a procedure, which, strangely enough, was advocated by a member of the Council. Fortunately the tendency was checked, and few, if any, cellars are occupied as separate dwellings at the present time.

Canal Boats used as Dwellings

An Act regulating canal boats used as dwellings was passed in 1877. The registration certificate issued under this Act to the master and owner defines the number of persons of each age and sex who may occupy the boat as a dwelling. A certificate identifying the number and lettering of the boat is also issued to the owner. The regulations provide for ventilation, amount of cubic space, separation of the sexes, and general healthiness and convenience of accommodation of the boat. Children dwelling on the boat are, for the purpose of the Elementary Education Acts, deemed to be resident in the place where the boat is registered.

In a further Act passed in 1884 certain additions were made to the previous Act which enabled the Local Government Board to make regulations with respect to school attendance and sanitary needs of those dwelling on the boat.

The only canal having direct communication with Liverpool is the Leeds and Liverpool Canal, the length of the waterway being about 3 miles. A great variety of cargoes is carried; many boats plying on the canal bring coal from the Wigan districts and return with manure or other offensive cargoes. All of these have been fitted with double bulkheads in conformity with the Act.

Year by year numerous changes have taken place in regard to the boats, old ones being broken up and new ones constructed. In 1879 there were 282 boats on the register, a number considerably increased as time went on; in 1900 there were 607. Notices are sent to the School Authorities when children are found living on canal boats, and not attending any school. These children are taken charge of by relatives and sent to school.

Certain boats plying on the canal but also plying on the Mersey have been registered with the Board of Trade and also under the Merchant Shipping Act. Difficulty arose as to their inspection as it was claimed that they were outside the jurisdiction of the Canal Boats Acts, but this difficulty was overcome by appointing the Canal Boat Inspectors as Port Sanitary Inspectors in 1898, and thus giving the inspectors the right to examine any boat. No doubt a similar difficulty existed in other ports, and in 1923 the Ministry of Health, which succeeded to the powers given to the Local Government Board by the 1884 Act, issued an order which brought all similar vessels hitherto registered under the Merchant Shipping Acts within the scope of the Canal Boats Acts, thus applying the Liverpool method of 1898 to all similarly placed districts.

Difficulties with canal boats used as dwellings are the same as those incidental to dwellings but complicated by the constantly moving population; sickness may be difficult to control, the education of children is a difficulty, and above all the question of childbirth in a habitation of this kind is one which does suggest the advisability of the expectant mother coming to hospital or some suitable place; this, no doubt, is usually done, but it is by no means always the case. Important as the question of education of children is, this latter question is of far more importance still.

The conditions of life are difficult but there are many circumstances which make life on a canal boat certainly as wholesome as in a city back street.

Of late years it has been found that families on boats on the canal had a home ashore in addition to that on board, and during the last ten years only two cases have been found in which there was not a home ashore.

The number of canal boats on the register has been considerably reduced, and in 1929 there were 352 boats.

Chapter IX

HOUSING OPERATIONS

Early vicious construction—"Courts"—Known later as "insanitary property"—Absence of building control—Inquiry and legislation—A "housing rate" not to exceed 1d. in the £ proposed—Method of procedure—Further legislation and method by presentment to the Grand Jury—Value of this procedure—New policy as to letting—Housing of the Working Classes Act, 1902—Arbitration—Cost of work to 1910—Licensed premises—Progressive procedure—Saving in cost of cleansing and sanitary supervision—Building in the outskirts—Churches, schools, playgrounds, shops, etcetera—Pre-war and post-war rents.

THE Rev. William Enfield in a history of Liverpool published in 1773 remarks: "The first observation which a stranger makes upon his arrival in Liverpool is generally that the streets are much too narrow, either for convenience or health. This is owing to the want of a regular plan of building, so that each builder builds in whatever place and form best suits his purpose". Dr Moss, in a Medical Survey of Liverpool addressed "to the inhabitants at large" in 1784, points out that the increasing commerce as well as the health of the town will suffer on account of the manner in which the buildings of the city are developing; houses too crowded together, streets too narrow in lay-out; and he suggests the widening of some of the existing congested streets, the expense of which would be met by the increased value of the new fronts on the improved streets when sold. Dr Moss' advice "to the inhabitants at large" had no effect.[1]

The seeds of future trouble were sown early; structural evils of the city accumulated with great rapidity and without check until the passing of the Liverpool Improvement Act of 1842, which, among its many useful clauses, imposed some restrictions upon the building of courts of the more vicious type, and gave some control over cellar dwellings, to which Dr Rutter, amongst others, had called attention. But meanwhile every open space in

---

[1] *Medical Survey of Liverpool*, by W. Moss, M.D. 1784.

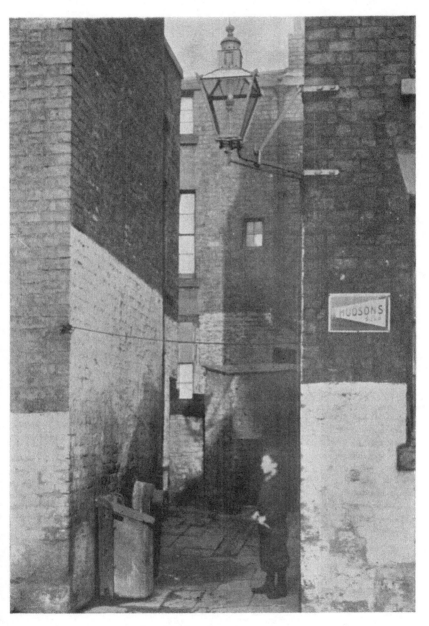

A unit of an insanitary area.

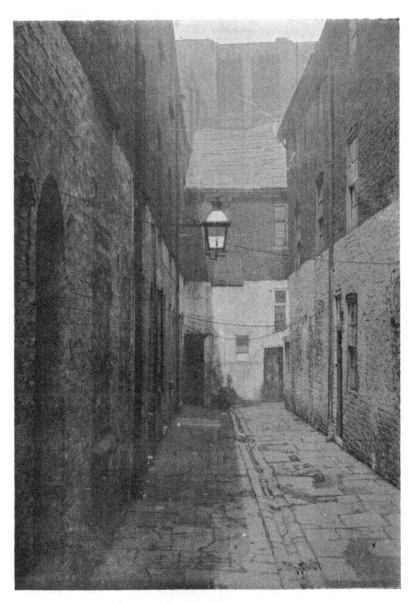

A unit of an insanitary area.

the districts occupied by the labouring classes had been covered
with houses consisting solely of three rooms one above the other,
placed in rows averaging six or eight, known as "courts", back to
back and side to side, frequently approached by a tunnel entrance,
9 or 10 feet separating the fronts of the opposite rows. The high
value of the land, increasing with the opportunity of builders
and landlords to exploit the needs of the rapidly growing population and secure the most profitable investment for their money,
resulted in complete disregard of elementary sanitary needs;
insufficient water supply and defective scavenging adding to the
miseries of the situation.

Typical examples are shown in the photographs. The "conveniences" were placed one at each side of one end of the court
and in full view of all the residents. A single tap placed in the
court was the only supply of water, and a box at the entrance
served as an ash-pit.

The term "insanitary property" became identified in Liverpool with this particular class of property, owing to the large
amount of it then existing and which accumulated during the
next twenty years. In 1864 there were upwards of 3000 courts,
and it is estimated that they represented not less than 22,000
insanitary houses of the type described.

So far as housing is concerned the application of the Improvement Act of 1842 was difficult, costly and slow in operation,
and it failed to stop the erection of houses of a highly undesirable
type. Some of those in responsible positions were alive to this
fact, but in the absence of a supporting public opinion the
advocacy of improvement not infrequently cost councillors their
seats in the Council—a phenomenon not wholly absent even
at the present day.

The continuance of this unhappy state of affairs, accompanied
by the excessive prevalence of disease and mortality, led the
Council in 1863 to appoint a Special Committee to review the
position in regard to the insanitary property which existed in
Liverpool, and, *inter alia*, to advance the introduction of the
water-carriage system into the courts. Apropos of this latter
recommendation the observations of Dr Trench, the then
Medical Officer of Health, are interesting, as showing the feeling

at the time: "The reform is one which will press heavily on individuals. Though the object which prompted their erection was selfish, unheeding cupidity, yet the present owners, being so by purchase, without the responsibility of the construction, may now plead the prescription of years, and very naturally object to improvements instituted and perfected solely at their expense". The purport of the recommendations was that the Town Council might with propriety assist the parties by affording them, at the public expense, the services of scavengers to supervise the water-carriage system, if, and when, it could be introduced in these courts.

The Special Committee also recommended amendments of the 1842 Act with a view to simplify, accelerate and cheapen procedure, and indeed took the then bold course of recommending that if necessary an additional rate for the purpose be obtained, *such rate not to exceed* 1*d. in the* £. They "feel confident that, by the judicious employment of a fund thus raised, the comfort and happiness of the poorer portion of the labouring class may be greatly promoted, much pecuniary loss to them from sickness and inability to work prevented, the public health improved, and the rate of mortality for the borough diminished".

The proposition resulted in the Liverpool Sanitary Amendment Act of 1864, but the halting use made of the measure was, for many years, virtually limited to the removal here and there of obstructive houses forming part of the worst type of court, and of courts in St Andrew Street and Trowbridge Street in proximity to the public slaughter-houses, "concerning which places, complaints and remonstrances have been sent to the Health Committee".[1]

The method of procedure under the Act may be summarised as follows:

1. The Medical Officer of Health shall report to the Council that certain houses (specifying them) are unfit for human habitation.

2. The Council, after approving the report, must send the same to the Clerk of the Peace, and notice of the report must be given to the owners of the properties included therein.

[1] See p. 197.

3. The report is then brought before the Grand Jury at Quarter Sessions, who, after hearing evidence and viewing the property, decide whether or not the houses mentioned in the report are insanitary and ought to be demolished. If they decide in favour of demolition, their doing so is called a "presentment".

4. The owners have a right of appeal to Quarter Sessions from the decision of the Grand Jury.

5. After presentment the properties may be acquired by agreement or by arbitration.

The Artisans' Dwellings Act of 1875 enabled a notoriously insanitary area known as the Nash Grove area (now renamed Victoria Square) to be dealt with as one in which the badly constructed courts and underground habitations predominated, and in which the provisions of the Act might most advantageously be applied; part of the area was rough unbuilt land upon which building was commenced with a minimum of inconvenience to the tenants of the insanitary section, who were transferred in due course until the whole area was dealt with. The buildings were completed and opened in 1885 by Mr Cross, the then Home Secretary and author of the Act. An extension followed subsequently.[1]

Owing to ill health Dr Trench was unable to carry on his duties and in 1876 Alderman Taylor vacated his position as Chairman of the Health Committee, which at that time dealt with housing problems, and was appointed Deputy Medical Officer, and shortly after succeeded Dr Trench as Medical Officer of Health. The Chairmanship of the Committee was filled by Sir Arthur Forwood, who stimulated an active campaign against insanitary property, a procedure which ultimately led to the appointment of a permanent committee under the title of Insanitary Property Committee in 1883.

Owing, amongst other reasons, to insufficiency of staff it cannot be said that the Act of 1864 was put to really effective use until 1883.[2] In that year, and in the large presentments subsequent to it, the individual owners of property and the

[1] See Table, page 172.
[2] About this time a philanthropic effort was made by Mr Philip Holt, by the purchase and demolition of certain highly insanitary courts, to stimulate municipal effort in this direction.

Liverpool Land and House-owners Association exercised their right to be represented before the Grand Jury at Quarter Sessions by counsel, and contest the presentments. The Corporation was represented for some years at the earlier of these inquiries by counsel who in after years attained great eminence, e.g. Mr Pickford, subsequently Lord Justice Pickford, Master of the Rolls, and Mr Walton, subsequently Mr Justice Walton. Some, amongst the array of counsel engaged on the other side, became no less distinguished in after life, as is evidenced by the fact that Mr F. E. Smith, a future Lord High Chancellor of England, was amongst the number.

The protracted arguments, the discussions, the sifting of evidence at these inquiries had valuable uses. At those times the truth of the terrible indictment against the insanitary areas was not realised either by Parliamentary or other Committees as it is now, the case now plain and generally admitted was not plain then, but inquiries and cross-examinations brought into prominence and established the facts which are no longer in question. The battles against slumdom were in fact fought and won then, and it is worth recording that in no single instance was medical evidence brought forward in opposition to the presentments.

Other, and perhaps more intelligible subjects of controversy, were the claims under the arbitration clause, as this dealt not only with houses but with business premises and profits from trade which in the case of licensed slum premises were very great; indeed the inclusion of three public-houses in the present-ment comprising the Hornby Street area involved as large a cost for their compensation alone, as the whole of the rest of the area. Incidents of this kind raised the question whether sums of money voted for housing could legally be applied to these purposes, and in order to avoid this cost several areas were subsequently reconstructed leaving the licensed premises un-touched, an unfortunate procedure which not only interfered with the scheme as a whole but left the demoralising influences of the public-house.[1]

On several occasions of the earlier presentments following

[1] See pp. 38 *et seq.*

1883, after the demolition of the insanitary property the sites were sold to builders, with a condition that they should erect thereon houses for the working classes, but no obligation was imposed as to the class of person to be accommodated or the rents to be charged. Very few of the former tenants of the demolished property were able to afford the rent charged for the new houses although in one case land was sold at 2*s*. 6*d*. per yard to a builder, the commercial value actually being about 35*s*. per yard.

For a number of years, virtually until 1895 or 1896, there were empty houses available in other districts, but their number gradually diminished, and in 1896 the position became so serious that the Council decided that the houses built to replace insanitary tenements should be let only to those who had been dispossessed, and in the year 1900, with a view to emphasising this position, the name of the committee which had been dealing with the demolition and clearance of insanitary property was changed from "Insanitary Property Committee" to "Housing Committee", and from that date strictly adhered to the policy of restricting the tenancy in the rehousing schemes to those dispossessed by the action of the Sanitary Authority.

It will be appreciated that it was neither desirable nor possible to rehouse the whole of the dispossessed population on the original site, bearing in mind the rapid increase in the numbers of a population of the character of those dealt with.

In the year 1902 the Corporation adopted the Housing of the Working Classes Act, 1890 (Part I), for the purpose of dealing in a more comprehensive manner with large unhealthy areas.

The procedure under Part I of this Act for clearing an insanitary area is as follows:

1. The Medical Officer of Health must make a report (or, as it is called in the Act, "an Official Representation") to the Council that a certain area, *considered as a whole*, is unhealthy, and can only be made sanitary by demolition and reconstruction.

2. If the Council is satisfied of the truth of the official representation, it must prepare an "improvement scheme", showing the area to be dealt with and the property to be demolished, with proper plans to illustrate the same.

3. The Council then proceeds to obtain a provisional order to acquire compulsory powers to obtain the properties included in the scheme.

4. The improvement scheme shall provide for the erection of such number of workmen's dwellings in place of those demolished as shall satisfy the Local Government Board.

The proceedings necessary to obtain the provisional order are to all intents and purposes the same as those taken to obtain powers to acquire land for street improvements or other purposes.

The Act remedied the disadvantages of the local Act, which did not provide for the compulsory purchase by the Corporation and compulsory sale by owners after arbitration, of properties other than insanitary dwellings. The consequence of these disabilities was that rebuilding might be obstructed unless the owners of obstructive buildings or sites were willing to sell, and, in the case of small areas, the Corporation was saddled with useless, isolated plots which became depositing grounds for rubbish and filth; a result of piecemeal procedure. Areas covered almost exclusively with insanitary property, and of sufficient size for reconstruction, were still to be found, and in these cases incidental questions of obstructive buildings, and so forth, were easily adjusted.

Between 1902 and 1910 three large areas were dealt with; one may be taken as an illustration, namely the Bevington Street area containing 295 houses, of which number 267 were insanitary, i.e. of the back-to-back type. The total contents of the area were 18,000 square yards, and the total cost £52,000 (including trade compensation), or £2.17s.9d. per yard. The new dwellings comprise 15 blocks containing 226 tenements, which provide for 1372 people. There are 52 self-contained cottages of five rooms each, 27 four-roomed, 70 three-roomed, and 77 two-roomed dwellings, together with a superintendent's house and office. Ample playgrounds are provided, and the demand for suitable shops is met by the provision of six shops at the main corners.

The "degradation" of an area originally laid out in a suitable manner is shown by the St Anne Street district, which in its first stage consisted of roomy houses with gardens and open spaces; the next stage, the complete conversion of the area into a compact nest of honeycomb slums of back-to-back houses built on these gardens and open spaces; the third stage, the entire demolition of these slums, clearance of the area, and the erection of sanitary dwellings on the site in 1913.

The periods for which loans were granted were eighty years in respect of land and sixty years in respect of buildings. The charge for interest and instalments of principal for the first year after the money was borrowed was £11,220. This sum was diminished annually by the proceeds of the investment of the annual instalments of the principal. This annual charge, however, was further reduced by the net receipts from the rents of the properties erected, which, based on the rents at that time fixed by the Committee, approximated to £3100 per annum. The net cost to the Corporation, therefore, on the total expenditure of £225,500 for the purchase of the sites and the erection of dwellings thereon, was equivalent to a little over ½d. in the £ on the rates at that time.

The total cost of the work of demolition and housing up to January 1, 1910, amounted to £980,739. Deducting the net rents of the dwellings from the charges for interest and sinking fund on the balance of debt leaves a sum of about £34,460, which amount was charged to the rates, and was equivalent to slightly over 2d. in the £.

The areas selected by the Housing Committee for the erection of dwellings were those which, up to the time of their demolition, were most notoriously insanitary. One of them, for example, the Adlington Street area, had figured prominently in every outbreak of infectious disease which had occurred in Liverpool; in each one of the great outbreaks of cholera and typhus fever it had been conspicuous.

It was confidently urged, *inter alia*, by the opponents of the work of the Housing Committee, that overcrowding would result from their operations, and it is noteworthy that actually the reverse has been the case. Year by year, and step by step, as the work proceeded the offence of overcrowding slowly diminished under the careful visitation and supervision of the staff of the Health Committee.[1]

In reporting upon the health of the city in 1912 the Medical Officer felt constrained to refer to the question of licensed premises upon insanitary areas, and to urge that in no instance should these premises be excluded in dealing with the areas. "He is fully aware that the cost of previous schemes has been greatly increased by the large amount of compensation paid for licensed premises, but at the same time the advantages to the district from the reduction of their numbers are so great that it would be a misfortune to depart from the previous practice." The Council has never had occasion to regret the adoption of this course in areas then conspicuous for their extreme squalor and poverty, and it is in these very areas that such large sums of money are expended in these premises. Indeed at a recent compensation inquiry counsel acting on behalf of one firm whose extensive ownership entitles its views to consideration, stated that a public-house in such a situation "is situated perhaps in the best neighbourhood for the public-house trade to be found in all Liverpool," and occupies "a particularly commanding position, and the people were of the right sort, from the publican's point of view, as customers". The plan of inclusion of these premises and paying compensation was reverted to.[2]

The term "insanitary property", as originally applied in Liverpool, it will be observed, referred solely to the mass of dwelling-houses built back-to-back and side-to-side in rows, a definition, although still retained, lacking in inclusiveness. The insanitary property in other towns was, broadly speaking, less vicious in original construction, consequently while in cities such as Birmingham, Manchester or Nottingham, structural alterations might afford adequate ameliorative measures, there was no such possibility with the old slums of Liverpool, for which one remedy, and only one, was possible—namely demolition.

There was, and still is, a large amount of property which is neither back-to-back nor side-to-side with similar houses, but with small back yards or back passages; it is, however, so

[1] See p. 168.   [2] See p. 38.

dilapidated, close and confined, and lacking in sanitary conveniences, as to be quite comparable with the insanitary property of the cities mentioned. This class of property, while not coming within the temporary definition as then applied in Liverpool, comprises some 6000 houses hardly removed from a justifiable inclusion in the term "insanitary property". A great deal of this class of property has been dealt with by improvements, but much more remains to be done.

Commercial developments have largely assisted in ridding the city of insanitary areas; they led to the clearance for business sites of areas previously covered with slum dwellings, increasing the value of the sites for business purposes, but lessening their suitability for dwellings, and at the same time adding to the numbers of dispossessed tenants for whom the City Council felt it its duty to provide, since ordinary builders did not care for this class of tenant, who were either unable or unwilling to pay a reasonable rental.

As long ago as 1869 the Corporation erected a block of 134 tenements known as St Martin's Cottages; these have from time to time been reconstructed and are still fully occupied. The year 1885 saw the opening of the Victoria Square Dwellings; five years later the block of labourers' dwellings erected in Juvenal Street, adjoining, was opened. These together contained 371 tenements to accommodate a total of 1382 people.

By the year 1893, 4126 insanitary houses had been demolished by the City Council at a total cost of £265,580, or an average cost of £64. 7s. per house, and about an equal number by railway and other commercial companies. Meanwhile 1062 dwelling-houses had been erected on the cleared areas giving accommodation for 5310 persons, but the displaced population probably exceeded those provided for by upwards of 10,000. Furthermore, a considerable number of houses had been erected by private builders on land sold for the purpose, and as the dispossessed tenants were not willing to pay an adequate rental for them, they were let in the usual course to any suitable tenant who applied.

For a time the policy of the Council to reserve for the dispossessed all houses erected on insanitary areas resulted in newly constructed houses remaining empty until rentals were reduced to a very low level.

Delays in rebuilding led to delays in slum clearances because it was feared that overcrowding would ensue in sub-let and other houses. The real danger, however, as pointed out in 1897, lay rather in the circumstance that these neglected hovels were falling into a condition of disrepair which rendered further habitation impossible. By lapse of time and by neglect the houses became structurally dilapidated, the internal woodwork defective, the plaster work bulged and perishing, and fouled by exhalations from the skin and lungs of occupants. Many, empty and derelict, were abandoned even by the poorest, and, as a consequence, areas which might with advantage be occupied by dwellings suitably planned for artisans, were encumbered with ruinous tenements obstructing light and ventilation, mere depositing grounds for rubbish, whilst their former tenants were shifting into sub-let houses of the lowest class in the vicinity.

The owners of this worn-out property did not give it attention; obviously there was only one real remedy, namely demolition; there were no doubt many remediable minor defects which the owners were loth to remedy even under the compulsion of statutory sanitary notices, regarding such measures as waste of money on a hopeless task. Yet the removal of these insanitary centres did not necessarily lead to overcrowding elsewhere, as the tendency to overcrowd the sub-let lodging-houses was kept in check by the Health Committee's staff.[1]

---

[1] The actual offences in this regard frequently arose not from want of space in the individual houses but from the overcrowding of all the tenants into one room; indeed rearrangement of the accommodation under the advice and supervision of the staff was resulting in a marked diminution of the offence, and at the close of the year 1897 the City Council, with the sanction of the Local Government Board and on the recommendation of the Health Committee, adopted amended byelaws which provided that "every lodger above 10 years of age shall have not less than 400 cubic feet of air space, and every person below 10 years of age shall have not less than 200 cubic feet, but if the room is used as a day-room as well as a bed-room, then every inmate must have at least 400 cubic feet". Under the then existing byelaws a space of 350 feet only was required, and two persons under twelve years were regarded as one adult.

One result of these byelaws—which required so relatively large an addition to the cubic space allowed for each lodger—was to put an entirely new definition upon the offence of overcrowding, and although the great majority of the people quickly appreciated the effect of the new byelaws, yet there

It was in this year (1897) that the Parks and Gardens Committee, with the desire to brighten the homes of the poorer citizens, distributed some thousands of flowering plants for window-boxes in the poorer quarters of the city. The attempt in the courts was not a success, and it was subsequently realised that "they were not suitable for growing plants, and although they have been frequently inspected with this object, they have been passed over each time for the same reason".

The sixteenth presentment (1899) finally disposed of the insanitary block—Bispham, Henry Edward, Adlington and Lace Street—which figured in every epidemic from Dr Duncan's time onwards and in which many temporary expedients short of demolition had been brought to bear. At this time the registration of all cellars let as separate dwellings was complete.[1]

In 1890 the Medical Officer prepared a permanent record showing the particulars of every court then existing in the city. This record was revised as the class of property diminished under (*a*) operation of the Insanitary Property Committee, (*b*) demolitions for extension of business premises, (*c*) demolition by the City Engineer or by the owners on account of danger of falling, 285 houses being dealt with in this category. In 1900 there still remained a total of 7431 houses coming within the limited definition of "insanitary" (as applied to houses which were back-to-back) in scattered groups under widely different conditions in regard to the areas in which they were situated. Closure under the Public Health Act was employed in isolated cases, whilst groups of houses were dealt with either under the Liverpool Sanitary Amendment Act, which enabled demolition to follow upon closure, or under the Housing of the Working

was temporarily an increase in the number of persons dealt with by the magistrate for disregarding the provisions of the byelaws.

Night inspections of sub-let houses and common lodging-houses for the purpose of detecting cases of overcrowding, or mixing of sexes, are carried on from year's end to year's end. The inspectors engaged upon this duty proceed in couples for the purpose of corroboration, and for protection in the rougher quarters of the city. In all cases a copy of the byelaws, and a notice indicating the number of persons who may occupy each room, are served upon the chief tenant, and these notices are renewed in the case of a new tenancy.

[1] See p. 153.

Classes Act, which afforded greater facilities in regard to removal of obstructive and objectionable buildings other than dwelling-houses, but in either case the procedure was defective and the question was raised during the year of obtaining further amendments to the Liverpool Act which would enable a still more rapid closure of these places to be effected, and this project met with acceptance.

The writer further emphasised his belief that the best interests of the labouring classes—those for whose benefit the work is undertaken—would be served by housing them, so far as circumstances will permit, in more open localities in the suburbs. Provision upon the original site or in the immediate vicinity had its limitations, and it was incorrect to assume that the occupants of congested insanitary areas were living near their work; as often as not they work at very considerable distances away. Projected advances in the means of locomotion between the centre of the city and the outskirts were designed to place within the reach of the working classes the advantages of living away from the congested centres of the city and yet within easy and cheap access of their work, wherever it may be, while the incidental benefits derived from removal from areas where the public-houses and their consequences were so obtrusively in evidence were not lost sight of.

The changed conditions in the habits and cleanliness of the people in areas which have been dealt with can only be appreciated by those who are conversant with the state of the localities prior to the operation of the Housing Acts. A walk round these improved districts during the day or night will indicate the atmosphere of quietness and comparative comfort which prevails, and the well-lighted rooms of the tenements present a cheerful appearance. The improvement extends beyond the immediate vicinity of the dwellings and affects the general condition of the neighbourhood; children are better clad and cared for, and there is a decrease or absence of police prosecutions for drunkenness and assault. There is a general feeling amongst the occupiers of the Corporation tenements that it is a privilege to dwell in them, and although in many cases they are among the poorest there is an evident endeavour to improve domestic conditions.

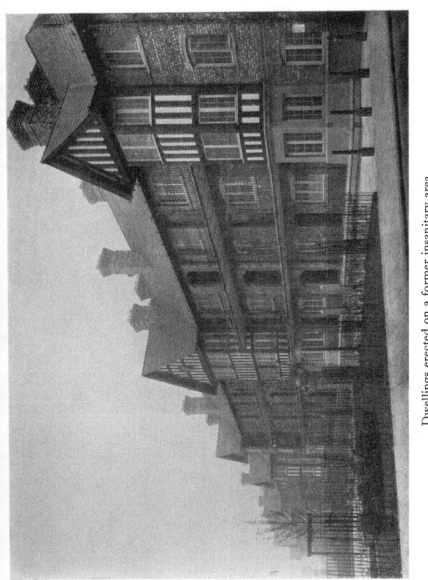

Dwellings erected on a former insanitary area.

The Medical Officer advised that persons selected for the position of caretaker of these tenements should be chosen from the type of tradesmen which usually supplied the class of Sanitary Inspectors, and should give evidence, such as is afforded by the possession of a Sanitary Certificate, of fitness and capacity to advise the tenants upon sanitary matters.

Quite apart from the improved health of those immediately concerned, the removal of insanitary property led to a great saving of the time of the officers of the Health Department hitherto occupied in efforts to ameliorate slum conditions, whose services are now available for duties in other directions.

It was estimated that by the removal of these courts there was a saving of upwards of £3000 per annum in the cost of cleansing and sanitary supervision alone.

The gradual decrease in the number of courts by demolition either for business requirements or by the action of the Housing Committee is shown by the number scheduled for daily supervision by the Sanitary Inspectors; in 1890 it was 2165, in 1895 it had fallen to 1660, in 1900 it was 1195, in 1905 it was 927, and in 1910 it was 604, showing a diminution in twenty years of 1561 courts and alleys, of which 323 were demolished during the five years 1906–10. The results in regard to individual houses dealt with up to January 1, 1910, under various Acts of Parliament may be conveniently seen as follows:

Number dealt with under the Liverpool Act of 1864 by presentment	6,344
Number dealt with owing to the demolition of certain houses to provide separate yard space, water supply and sanitary accommodation for surrounding houses	about 1,500
Demolished for trade and other purposes by private enterprise	about 5,600
Number dealt with by various Improvement Schemes under the Housing of the Working Classes Act since 1902 .	1,720
	Total 15,164
Number which the Medical Officer of Health reported as existing on January 1, 1910	4,150

The dates of the various presentments under the Liverpool Act of 1864 and the numbers of houses dealt with by each are as follows:

	Year			Total
1st presentment	1864	included	85 houses ⎫	
2nd ,,	1865	,,	104 ,,	
3rd ,,	1865	,,	189 ,,	
4th ,,	1868	,,	73 ,,	625
5th ,,	1871	,,	85 ,,	
6th ,,	1880	,,	89 ,, ⎭	
7th ,,	1884	,,	359 ,, ⎫	
8th ,,	1884	,,	690 ,,	
9th ,,	1889	,,	119 ,,	2200
10th ,,	1890	,,	533 ,,	
11th ,,	1891	,,	499 ,, ⎭	
12th ,,	1894	,,	577 ,, ⎫	
13th ,,	1896	,,	240 ,,	
14th ,,	1897	,,	890 ,,	
15th ,,	1898	,,	365 ,,	3519
16th ,,	1899	,,	706 ,,	
17th ,,	1901	,,	369 ,,	
18th ,,	1904	,,	372 ,, ⎭	
				Total 6344

The action under other Acts of Parliament is alluded to elsewhere, but the numbers of tenements erected on the old insanitary areas up to the War are conveniently shown as follows:

Situation	Opened in	Total No. of Tenements
St Martin's Cottages	(1869)	124
Victoria Square	(1885)	282
Juvenal Dwellings	(1890)	102
Arley Street	(1897, 1902–3)	46
Gildart's Gardens	(1897, 1904)	229
Dryden Street	(1901)	182
Kempston Street	(1902)	79
Kew Street	(1902)	114
Adlington Street Area	(1902–3)	272
Hornby Street Area	(1904, 1906–7)	455
Eldon Street	(1905)	12
Stanhope Cottages	(1904)	60
Mill Street	(1904)	55
Clive Street and Shelley Street	(1905)	83
Upper Mann Street	(1905–6)	88
Combermere Street	(1909)	49
Burlington Street	(1910)	114
Saltney Street	(1911)	48
Grafton Street	(1911)	60
Bevington Street	(1912)	224
Northumberland Street	(1913)	68
St Anne Street	(1914)	78
Gore Street	(1916)	24
Jordan Street	(1916)	31
Sparling Street	(1916)	16

Total 2895
including 79 self-contained
cottages and 32 shops

It will be generally conceded that great success has resulted from the planning of the environs of the city well in advance, largely owing to the prevision and successful advocacy of Mr Brodie, the late City Engineer, and the enlightened views of the Health Committee and the Council. With a view to avert the danger to the rapidly growing city of a continued development upon the evil lines of the past, a special Improvement Committee had been appointed by the Council as long ago as 1859, and a carefully considered scheme for the construction of two concentric boulevards, an inner and an outer, was submitted by Mr Newlands, the then City Engineer. Mr Newlands comments on the uselessness of the trifling ameliorative measures which were hitherto adopted, and the advantages of the scheme: "Peddling improvements to abate small local imperfections are not only worthless, but become superannuated before they are carried into effect. It is only by a comprehensive scheme for the remedy of present evils, and the preventing their repetition, and by providing for future requirements, that any plan of improvement really worthy of consideration can be made". Mr Newlands pointed out the facilities which such a project would afford for obtaining land for parks and playgrounds, "while the boulevard in itself would fulfil the conditions of being a healthy place of resort for the people....It would truly be an elongated park passing through a country affording ever-varying and charming prospects". More than half a century elapsed before principles of this character were fully put into operation.

The inner boulevard, easy of access, "would possess more immediately the advantages of a sanitary cordon, and by changing the whole character of the locality, prevent to a great extent the huddling together of the wretched streets and mean houses which are so rapidly springing up in the outskirts of the town".

The advantages of such a development, with appropriate streets leading into them, were manifest, but the proposals were not approved; had the recommendations found favour the whole course of the sanitary history of Liverpool would have been changed, and large sums subsequently expended in undoing consequent mischief would have been saved.

Mr Newlands' forecast so far as the outer boulevard is concerned has been realised to a remarkable degree by the action of Mr Brodie, and those acting with him; it is of great interest to sketch the lines of the boulevards proposed by Mr Newlands, the inner of which has been closely built over, with a large proportion of slum property, the outer approximating to the lines subsequently adopted by Mr Brodie in the construction of the Queen's Drive.

The cost of the outer boulevard, together with the accessories suggested, was estimated by Mr Newlands at £14,200, and that of the inner boulevard at £14,700; the suggested improvements in existing streets naturally reached a much higher figure.

Projects similar in principle, but smaller in scale, had indeed already been put forward; some of the main roads leading out of Liverpool to the north were projected in 1847, some were proceeded with and to-day form the main arteries through Bootle. Lines of roads, no doubt modest in their conception, were then projected connecting Wavertree and West Derby. Within the town, improved accesses to the Pierhead, "the filling-up of St George's Dock Basin, and converting the area so obtained into a grand square or place, the removal of the Goree Warehouses and setting back of St Nicholas' Church-Yard," were proposed by Mr Newlands.... "It is assumed as a preliminary that the ground is cleared by the removal of the Goree Piazzas", a "preliminary" not yet given effect to, although St Nicholas' Churchyard was dealt with 48 years ago, as shown in the illustrations.

To-day skeleton plans are well laid out in advance and the subsequent building presents a very much simpler problem than that which arises in the difficult and costly task of reconstruction of old areas, a fact which helped very greatly in meeting the grave housing conditions at the close of the War.

The complete cessation of building during and for almost two years subsequent to the War accentuated the needs of the people in regard to housing and placed an entirely new complexion upon the obligations of the City Council. Difficulties were further added to by strikes in the building trade and lack of available labour, while large bodies of men, able and apparently willing to undertake work which would meet the public neces-

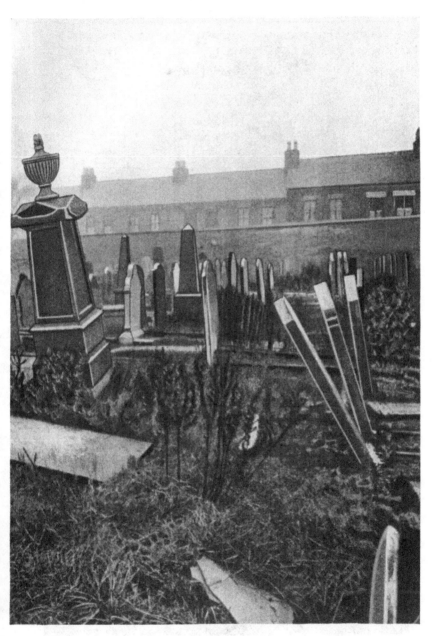

An old graveyard.

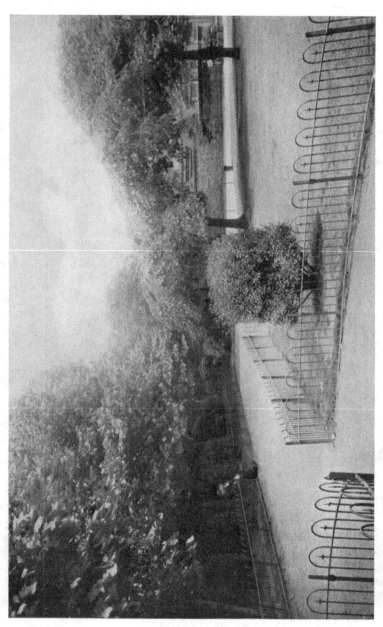

A town garden, formerly the burial ground shown in preceding illustration.

sities, were from lack of organisation unable to assist. For five years preceding the War private building enterprise had provided approximately 2000 dwelling-houses in Liverpool annually; the cessation of building for six years meant a deficit of some 12,000 new houses. Private enterprise, which had hitherto played so prominent a part in the building of small houses, was dead, grave labour difficulties were added, and a heavy and exacting burden was thrown upon the City Council.

The conditions brought serious discomfort to almost all classes of the community and resulted in overcrowding and sub-letting of a highly undesirable character, constituting a grave menace to the physical welfare of the people.

The first post-war Housing Act of Parliament, that of 1919, enabled a start to be made by the purchase of some 500 of the military huts at Knotty Ash Camp; their conversion provided temporary housing accommodation of 488 dwellings by the end of the year 1920.

Various Housing Acts followed, viz. 1923, 1924, and finally, during the Ministry of Mr Neville Chamberlain, the important Housing Act of 1925, which consolidated practically all enactments relating to the Housing of the Working Classes Acts in England and Wales.

Under these various Acts great work has been achieved, and in carefully selected parts of the outer areas of Liverpool a total of 2532 acres of land has been acquired, representing nearly four square miles, an area considerably larger than that of the adjoining borough of Bootle, and involving the construction of approximately 40 miles of roads and sewers. On these areas 13,560 houses and tenements and 56 shops have so far been erected, entirely constructed in brick-work.[1]

On the Norris Green Estate (the largest) six churches and seven Council schools have been erected, and provision is made for public baths, welfare centres, branch libraries, recreation grounds, billiard hall and other recreative buildings. In the planning of all the schemes wide arterial roads are provided and the natural features of the estates preserved as far as possible, and under the guidance of the Tramways Committee, with the

---

[1] For types and rentals, see pp. 176–7.

advice of Mr Priestley, a very adequate transport provision is made, all of the areas being served by direct lines of electric tramway, omnibus, rail, or all three.

Enough has been said to make it clear that the continuance of the work of reconstruction of central insanitary areas was by no means lessened, and upon the motion of the late Sir Archibald Salvidge the City Council in 1926 re-affirmed the provision that "the people dispossessed be rehoused as far as possible in the same area from which they had been dispossessed, and on the same principle of rents as in the past and in agreement with the Ministry of Health".

The City Council has decided that no part of the building estates shall be let for the erection of licensed premises.[1]

The houses built are of two types, "A" and "B", the accommodation of the former consisting of a large living room, scullery, three bedrooms, bathroom, larder, coal place and w.c. The "B" type house is similar, but is provided with a parlour in addition. Ample cupboard and shelving accommodation is provided, together with a linen cupboard, and in the living rooms of some of the houses a most useful dresser. Electric light is available in all the houses. Gas is laid on for cooking and heating, gas fires being fixed in the parlour and two bedrooms. Ample garden space is provided and facilities given for the erection of sheds, greenhouses, poles in connection with wireless apparatus, etcetera.

As much variety as possible has been introduced in the elevations, and considering the limitations imposed by the high cost of building, many pleasing exteriors have been achieved which bear favourable comparison with the best that has been done in any other part of the country.

As a general rule the type of plan selected was always dependent upon the aspect of the house. It was laid down as an essential that the living room of each house should get direct sunlight for some period of the day. In letting the houses preference was given to ex-service applicants, and those with large families.

Under the provisions of the Housing Act, 1919, a total of 84 houses were erected by private enterprise, whilst under

[1] See p. 166.

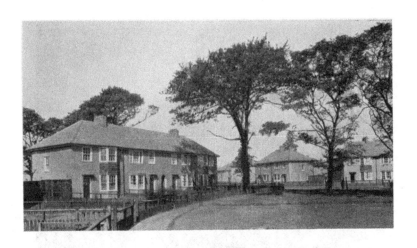

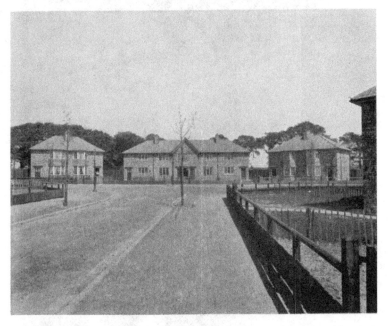

Types of houses erected on Norris Green Estate, showing wide road and open space.

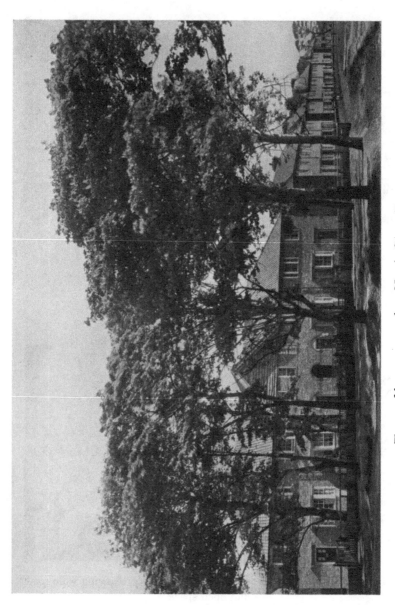

Types of houses erected on Norris Green Estate.

PRE-WAR RENTS OF TENEMENTS AND HOUSES

Pre-war tenements Composition rates		Gross per week s. d.	Nett per week s. d.	Houses	Gross per week s. d.	Nett per week s. d.
One-roomed	Ground floor	3 8	2 11	Cottages (self-contained)	8 11	6 11
	First	2 11½	2 4			
	Second	2 8	2 2	Four-roomed	10 6½	8 2
Two-roomed	Ground	5 4	4 2			
	First	4 5½	3 5			
	Second	4 2	3 3		13 8½	10 0
Three-roomed	Ground	6 9½	5 3			
	First	6 10½	4 8			
	Second	4 2	3 3			
Four-roomed	Ground	8 2	6 4			
	First	7 5	5 10			
	Second	7 2	5 7			

POST-WAR RENTS OF TENEMENTS AND HOUSES

Post-war tenements	Gross per week s. d.	Nett per week s. d.	Houses ("A" Non-parlour type) Gross per wk. s. d.	Nett per wk. s. d.	("B" Parlour type) Gross per wk. s. d.	Nett per wk. s. d.
Living room, two bedrooms, bathroom and scullery						
Ground floor	8 3	6 6	12 6	8 9	16 6	11 0
First ,,	7 9	6 1	13 6	9 9	17 3	11 6
Second ,,	7 6	5 11				
Living room, three bedrooms and scullery						
Ground floor	9 3	7 3	14 3	10 3	18 3	12 0
First ,,	8 9	6 10			19 3	13 6
Second ,,	8 9	6 8			(with special amenities)	

those of the Housing Act, 1923, the Corporation offered a lump sum subsidy of £75 per house to private enterprise builders to encourage the erection of houses, and also offered financial assistance to owner-occupiers in the acquisition of these houses under conditions approved by the Ministry of Health. This lump sum subsidy was subsequently reduced to £50 per house, and ceased on October 1, 1929. A total of 4274 of these houses has been completed and earned the subsidy.

In the new tenements erected at Melrose Road, some of them five storeys in height, two and three bedrooms are provided, with living room, scullery, separate w.c., bathroom and hot water system.

A large central area improvement scheme is being proceeded with which will involve the opening up or reconstruction of a large part of some seven acres. The most pressing part of the work is being proceeded with but certain legal difficulties have still to be overcome.

In clearances of insanitary areas playgrounds have been provided wherever possible—in many cases one for boys and another for girls; gymnasium appliances are also fitted in each. Side streets of short lengths are closed to vehicular traffic by posts, thus protecting children from this risk.

At the present time the approximate number of dwelling houses, tenements, and flats under maintenance by the Council reaches 21,726, housing well over 100,000 people.

The results of procedure in the outer areas are indicated in the following illustrations.

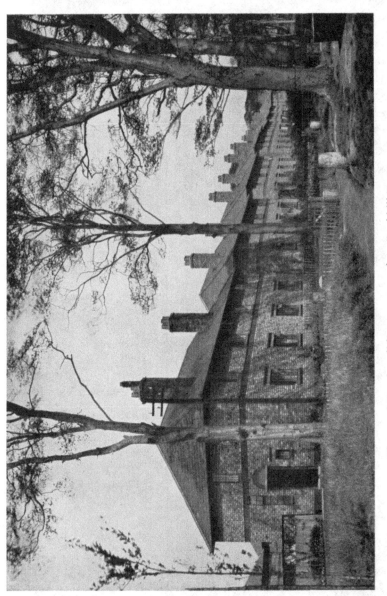

Types of "parlour" houses erected on Larkhill Estate.

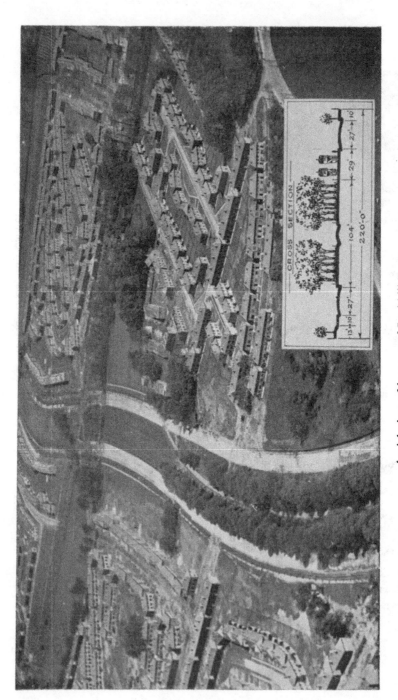

Aerial view of lay-out of Larkhill Estate.

Chapter X

MUNICIPAL CLEANLINESS

Scavenging and cleansing—Paving and sewering—Disposal of refuse.

Scavenging and Cleansing

IN the earlier record of civic administration references to cleansing and scavenging the town are few. Although the importance of the subject was not appreciated, provisions were made at an early date in the town's history to deal with obvious nuisances arising in the ill-paved and ill-constructed thoroughfares. It was customary in early times to require every carter after emptying his vehicle of the produce or materials he had brought into the town, to fill up his cart with rubbish before leaving, and so some portion of the town's refuse was removed without cost to the inhabitants.

It may be assumed that in those early times the inhabitants were responsible for the cleanliness of their own frontages. In the records for 1704 we read of the prosecution of two rectors for not cleansing the street before their barn in Dale Street, and the prosecution of an alderman for not cleansing the street before his own door and house, and at the "Grand Portmoot Court" held on October 23, 1721, it was ordered: "that the Bellman give public notice every Saturday night for every person to clean their Streets on pain of 3/4".

The Liverpool Sanitary Amendment Act of 1849 marked the beginning of a definite recognition of the importance of scavenging and cleansing. Owners of property were hitherto required to provide receptacles for refuse and for its removal at their own cost, but the Sanitary Act imposed this latter obligation upon the Council and a staff was appointed for the purpose.

In the year 1848, Mr James Newlands, the first Borough Engineer of Liverpool, drew attention to the type of boulder paving then existing in all but the most important thoroughfares of the town and urged the reconstruction of those streets as an essential factor towards their thorough cleansing. In the narrow streets not subjected to traffic and inhabited by the poorer population the evil was accentuated, for in the absence of a drainage system and proper conveniences the inhabitants threw a great deal of their refuse on the streets and brushing failed to remove it.

The extended powers in the Liverpool Act of 1842 had facilitated the completion of the work of sewering, but meanwhile, owing to the rapid growth of the population in the interval, the sewers when completed were insufficient for their purpose, and in order to avoid the cost of their necessary enlargement Parliamentary powers were obtained to prohibit newly constructed houses from draining into them,[1] a prohibition which resulted in the construction of thousands of pits and deep open channels for drainage and refuse, the solid part of which was carted away at variable intervals, the liquid oozing into the porous sandstone rock—the source indeed from which the water supply of the town was obtained. These pits and channels frequently extended from one end of the street to the other, and remained sources of injury to the town for many years, indeed they were not entirely abolished until the early 'nineties. Their condition may be gauged from the fact that their contents remained undisturbed from June till October, because experience showed that any attempt to empty them during the summer months invariably resulted in outbreaks of disease, notably the cholera of infants. However good, therefore, the system of sewers may have been for the limited population for which it was designed, the inadequacy of the scheme proved an injury to the growing town.

With regard to paving and flagging, the claims of the evergrowing slum areas, courts and alleys, absorbed more attention than the main thoroughfares.

The Act of 1846 enabled the Council either to employ direct labour in cleansing streets and removing refuse from dwellinghouses or to employ contractors. Up to the end of 1866 the Council followed the latter procedure, the work being carried

---

[1] At the same Session of Parliament another town applied for and obtained powers to compel owners to drain all newly constructed houses into the newly constructed sewers.

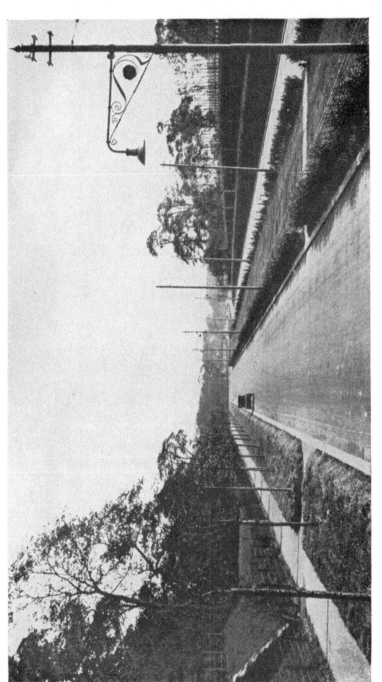

Menlove Avenue. New road and means of transport to new area.

out under the supervision of four inspectors in the pay of the Council.

There existed in the town huge middens in the form of long tunnels often extending beneath whole streets of houses filled for many months at a time with objectionable material of all descriptions. These were only emptied when the farmers required supplies of manure, so that when agriculturists were busily engaged at seed time and harvest there was no demand for these deposits and the night soil contractor was at a loss to find an outlet for the constantly accumulating refuse. Thus the community were forced to live in close proximity to the most abominable conditions for long periods at a time with the consequent menace to health.

In 1847 the Council had commenced an extensive sewerage system and instead of prohibiting (as had been the practice) all connections between privies and drains, began to compel such communication to be made. Water closets were also allowed to be discharged into the sewers, and newly built houses were supposed to be provided with such closets; the sewers however proved inadequate for dealing with the sewerage of newly built houses.

It was the end of 1860 before a proper system of water closet accommodation could be insisted upon and in 1863 the powers under the 15th section of the Liverpool Sanitary Amendment Act of 1854 were put into force and cesspools in situations prejudicial to health scheduled for conversion into water closets.

In 1866 the Council decided, not without opposition, to take over the immediate control of all cleansing operations, and to carry out this work by its own workmen.

In order to carry out the work, large stables and workshops were erected in different parts of the town and a number of houses purchased; wharves were erected on the banks of the Leeds and Liverpool Canal, adjoining the then Lancashire and Yorkshire Railway, and five other wharves were rented.

It is difficult to-day to realise the condition of affairs existing at that time when there were within the built-up portion of the city not less than 64,000 tons of night soil, awaiting removal, a prolific source of atmospheric pollution and breeding of flies.

Until the end of 1870 dry ash-pit refuse and the sweepings from the little-used macadam roads were conveyed to exhausted stone quarries and clay pits near by, but as building development proceeded complaints began to be made against the practice of building houses upon land which had been raised and levelled in this way. The report by Drs Parkes and Burdon-Sanderson, already alluded to,[1] resulted in restrictions being imposed upon this method of disposal of refuse.

Meanwhile difficulties were arising in regard to refuse containing too much organic matter for disposal by tipping, and too little to be of value to farmers as a fertiliser. In 1875 experiments by way of incinerators were undertaken by Mr George F. Deacon, the then Borough Engineer, and upon the recommendation of the then Chairman of the Health Committee, Sir Arthur Forwood, a system of disposal at sea by steam hopper barges, specially designed by Messrs Simons of Renfrew for that purpose, was inaugurated in 1876. These vessels were required to signal the lightship, 21 miles out, before discharging.

Before this could be brought into operation the huge quantities being dealt with at both Carr Hall Farm (near Burscough) and Bromborough Pool aroused the hostility of the rural authorities in these respective neighbourhoods, and opposition was demonstrated to such an extent that depositing on Carr Hall Farm was abandoned in 1875 and the Bromborough Pool in 1878.

A selection of the material had to be made at the wharves in order that products which could be economically disposed of to farmers, or others, should be separated from refuse destined for the sea, and to pick out rope and matting which would possibly entangle the chains operating the hopper floors.

By 1890 the quantity of refuse had increased beyond the powers of the existing systems of disposal, fogs and storms interfering with sea disposal during the winter months, and after some consideration it was decided that the lighter materials should be disposed of by burning. In 1891 the then City Engineer, Mr John A. Brodie, designed and erected at the Charters Street depot the first destructor for the purpose, originally designed to consume some six tons of refuse per cell

[1] See p. 99.

in twenty-four hours, a total of sixteen cells being ultimately in operation. Similar installations to meet the needs of other parts of the city were made in due course.

Meanwhile improvements were undertaken in connection with the cleansing of the streets. Up to 1891 the method of cleansing the main thoroughfares was by horse-drawn brushes at night, preceded by water-sprinkling, although water for this purpose was restricted until after July 1891, when water was available from Vyrnwy, and an important decision was made by the Health Committee to allow water to be used for flushing the streets, courts, etcetera, a project warmly espoused by Alderman John Houlding.

In 1895, the year of a large extension of the city's boundaries, it was decided to abolish all ash-pits and substitute bins to allow of a weekly collection of refuse to be loaded direct into the waiting vehicles, instead of the cumbersome monthly system which involved depositing the contents of the ash-pit temporarily upon the street.

In 1898 the whole of the cleansing and scavenging operations were placed under the supervision of Mr J. A. Brodie. Under his guidance small bins were employed in all new dwelling-houses, which greatly simplified the collection and removal of domestic refuse.

The clinker produced as a result of the establishment of the destructors was utilised for the purpose of the manufacture of concrete slabs, and the heat produced in the destructor was first used in 1900 for generating power for the electric tramway and lighting.

By the year 1921 post-war housing programmes were being carried into effect and, notwithstanding the high costs of building, developments on the municipal housing areas were rapid and the area to be covered by the Cleansing Department correspondingly increased.

The gradual abolition of ash-pits and substitution of bins made collection of refuse at night-time unnecessary, and a considerable economy ensued.

The phases in the development of municipal cleansing, already outlined, lead up to the important present-day operations of the

Cleansing Department, for which Mr Frank, the City Engineer, is responsible, and which meet the needs of a population approaching a million, an area of over 608 miles of streets with approximately 177,000 houses, besides shops, factories, and other premises. Some 1200 men are employed on this work and the city is equipped with depots, store yards, repair shops, stables and destructors, besides hopper barges.

As in other towns, the quantity of refuse collected per head of the population is still unduly high and appeals to the public are continually being made to burn more refuse, and so materially to reduce the cost of the work.

Efforts are constantly being made to improve the service in all its aspects, and investigations are pursued wherever there appears reasonable prospects of success by trying suggested new methods, e.g. the use of modern motor vehicles which, having a particularly low loading line, reduce the strain upon the workmen in lifting the bins, lessen the time taken in handling the refuse, and reduce the cost of transport.

Manure is removed from stable yards as often as required free of charge; this material is the favourite breeding place of flies, the frequent carriers of disease—a fact suggestive of the sanitary advantages of substitution of motor for horse traffic.[1] Paper suitable for pulping is collected periodically by arrangement with the Salvation Army, and, in view of the charitable nature of this organisation, the Corporation has not deemed it desirable to enter into competition. At present all clinker is used for road-making or other purposes, and is a source of revenue to the Department; 41,000 tons were sold during the municipal year 1926–7, and during the same period 4,230,000 units of electricity were generated with machinery operated by refuse destructor steam.

Tipping of suitable material is now being carried out in areas within the city for the purpose of filling up hollows and depressions on waste land and making such land suitable for recreation purposes; the system is to tip in layers of not more than 6 feet, and as the work proceeds the refuse is covered with a layer of earth and afterwards used for agricultural purposes,

[1] See Professor Newstead's Report, *Flies and their breeding places.*

or sown with grass seed and used as a playground. Since this method was adopted complaints have been practically eliminated, with a reduction of about 750 tons per week in the amount of refuse to be disposed of by burning. Pits and hollows on farm-land outside the city, served by canal barges or motor wagons, are similarly used, and the land reclaimed for agricultural purposes.

All main roads in the centre of the city receive constant attention throughout the day-time, a staff of orderly boys being engaged on this work.

With regard to the actual cost of the street cleansing and scavenging operations, and the disposal of domestic and other refuse, the estimates for the current year amount to £364,000, against which are sales of manufactured paving material and electrical energy, etcetera, of £19,000.

Chapter XI

CONTROL OF FOOD SUPPLIES

*Control of imported foodstuffs—Failure of Adulteration Act of
1872—Sale of Food and Drugs Act (1875) and Amendments—
Bacteriological analysis—Shell-fish—Tuberculosis and milk—
Arsenic in beer—Supervision of meat and other foodstuffs.*

To a City Council such as that of Liverpool, which is also
the Port Sanitary Authority, there falls a double duty in
respect of the supervision of food supplies, viz. that in connection with materials intended for local consumption, and also
such investigations of imported foodstuffs destined for other parts
of the country as may be necessary to safeguard prospective
consumers. The gradually widening knowledge of the causes and
consequences of unsoundness or adulteration of foodstuffs has
led to progressive legislation which has enabled measures to be
taken to deal with accidents or unforeseen difficulties affecting
the transport of food, as well as with the perverse ingenuity of
the fraudulent.

The Adulteration Act of 1872 provided penalties for the
wilful admixture of injurious or poisonous ingredients with any
article of food or drink; a penalty was also imposed for the
sale, as unadulterated, of any article of food or drink which
was adulterated. The 1872 Act further empowered the local
authority to appoint a competent chemical analyst for the purpose
of making analyses. Dr Campbell Brown, whose services had
already been called upon by the Water Committee, was appointed
to the post of City Analyst in 1872, nothing hitherto having been
done in this direction towards protecting the consumer. The
Council, no doubt with an eye to economy, resolved "that no
instruction for any analysis, the cost of which will exceed £1, be
given without the approval of the Finance Sub-Committee".
No machinery nor staff existed for the purpose of procuring
samples officially, the onus being left with the public, who were
informed through the press that any person sending a suspected
article could have it analysed, the name and address of the
sender being given as a necessary precaution against malicious

and vexatious complaints. If the analysis showed the *injurious* admixture, a further sample was to be taken from the same shop, and if that also showed *injurious* adulteration the matter was to be taken to court.

During the first six months in which the law was in operation eight samples were taken, three of them were milk and were reported as sour, deficient in cream, and adulterated with water, the peculiar taste of one of them being attributed to 30 per cent. of added water and the condition of the cans. A sample of water from a cistern contained a deposit of oxide of iron, lime salts and a trace of lead; a sample of bread is recorded to contain neither alum, plaster of paris, nor arsenic, which suggests the nature of the impurities which the analyst suspected.

The work of an inspector who was subsequently authorised to procure samples was hampered by the restriction temporarily imposed upon him: "no shop, and no article offered for sale, is to be treated as suspected unless complaint has been made by some person, and the good faith of the complainant guaranteed by his name and address...", and Dr Trench felt "that it would be most impolitic and most hurtful to leave an arbitrary discretion in this matter to any Inspector, however respectable and trustworthy....No Inspector, and indeed no Officer, however high his position, should be allowed to throw broadcast the slur of suspicion over any section, however humble, of the trading community".

It is not surprising that the 1872 Act became a dead letter, and, three years later, public health problems having in the meantime received the close attention of the Government, a further Act, the Sale of Food and Drugs Act, 1875, became law; it supplied many omissions in the Act which it superseded and enabled steps to be initiated to protect the consumer from injurious or other adulterations and frauds, by providing a penalty for selling to the prejudice of the purchaser any article which was not of the nature, quality and substance of the article asked for; it gave powers to the Council to appoint inspectors to purchase for analysis suspected articles of food, and the protection of traders from dishonest competition is an outcome of the Act.

It is upon this Act, and the many subsequent additions from time to time made to it, that the present efficient system of analysis of articles of food and drink and drugs is based.

For many years after the passing of the Act the use of chemical preservatives was exceedingly common, and in the case of readily perishable articles, such as milk, cream, etcetera, the addition of preservatives took the place of care and cleanliness, a procedure which no doubt checked putrefactive changes but at the same time lessened, or even destroyed, the value of the material by interference with the process of digestion. Boracic acid, or borates, and salicylic acid, or salicylates, were used indiscriminately for a number of years, the actual quantity found in different samples of the same foodstuff varying very widely, showing a loose method of use of the preservative.

Prosecutions were undertaken in these cases, and the defence usually took the form of claiming that the chemicals employed were commonly used by doctors as drugs, and that the purchaser of the article had the incidental advantage of a dose of physic without additional cost. Indeed medical evidence was given in court to prove the medicinal virtues of the preservative employed.

The use of colouring matter was so free that when the practice in regard to milk was arrested general complaints were received from the public, who regarded the yellow colour as the index of richness and purity, and the vendor had difficulty in persuading the customer that this was not the case; of all articles in which the use of chemical preservative is liable to be attended with mischief milk is the most likely.

Various Departmental and other Committees were appointed from time to time to consider these questions, and in 1899, when these practices were still rife and to an extent sanctioned by law, the writer advised a Departmental Committee to require that:

Every person adding any colouring matter or preservative whatever to articles of food should state on a plain label:
　　1. The material used.
　　2. The quantity used.
　　3. The date at which the material was added.

The advice was not accepted at the time but in later years the reports of Government Committees led to more effective legislation under the title of the Public Health (Preservatives in Food) Regulations, 1926.

The protection afforded to the public by the *chemical* examination of foodstuffs, and the extremely valuable results of that protection, paved the way to the adoption of means by which contamination of foodstuffs by living organisms could be detected and consequent mischief averted, e.g. typhoid infection by oysters or other shell-fish, tubercle infection by milk, or the changes giving rise to food poisoning, were among the points upon which bacteriological investigation was necessary.

An opportunity arose for pursuing this line of investigation by the appointment of Professor Rubert Boyce to the George Holt Chair of Pathology (of which Bacteriology formed an important branch) in 1894. The following year at the request of the writer Professor Boyce very readily undertook to make a number of investigations on the lines indicated, an early instance of the friendly co-operation which has so uniformly characterised the relationship of the university and the city. These examinations were carried on for several years without remuneration, but in 1897 cases of bacterial contamination were detected in which preventive legal measures could be instituted only through the certificates of an analyst appointed under the Sale of Food and Drugs Act of 1875. At the time of the passing of that Act, bacteriological research was not contemplated, consequently in order to clothe the Bacteriological Analyst with powers similar to those of the Chemical Analyst, it became necessary to satisfy the Local Government Board that Professor Boyce did possess adequate chemical knowledge. No difficulty arose in this matter, and the Local Government Board welcomed the new step which the City Council contemplated. The appointment of Professor Boyce as City Bacteriologist in 1897, warmly espoused by Alderman Cookson, was the first to be made in this country.

In due course bacteriological methods were applied to the investigation of a very wide range of subjects, including contamination of milk, cream, fish, tinned meats, and ice cream. The method was applied to investigations of infectious diseases, actual or suspected, in man and animals, such for example as diphtheria or tubercle in man, and anthrax or plague in animals, plague in the rat being of international importance in connection with shipping.[1] Arrangements were made by the Health Committee to enable examination in any case of infectious disease to be undertaken for medical practitioners in the city without any cost to them. The system has proved to be of great advantage in helping early diagnosis, and in the discovery of many unsuspected cases of infection.

Upon the death of Professor Boyce in 1911 a separate Chair of Bacteriology was established at the University with which the duties of the City Bacteriologist were associated, and Professor Beattie was appointed to these posts. The magnitude of the operations of the present highly organised City Bacteriological Department may be gauged by the fact that 38,412 samples were investigated during the year 1929, a number which includes the systematic daily analysis of samples of water taken from various points of delivery within the city.

Legislative powers being deficient, difficulty was experienced in giving the public protection from disease known to be derived from shell-fish taken from filth-polluted and unsuitable waters—frequently sewage-washed from their proximity to sewers constructed subsequent to the establishment of oyster beds or layings of other shell-fish.

Following upon bacteriological investigations a series of important recommendations were made in 1898 to the effect (1) that legislative measures should restrict the licensing of oyster beds, (2) that the trade should themselves form an association in order to provide for periodic examination of the layings, (3) that similar measures should be taken in reference to oysters imported from abroad, or the deposit of imported oysters in our own waters, (4) that there should be periodic inspection of gathering grounds of mussels, cockles, periwinkles, and adequate provision made for analyses.

With the authority of the Local Government Board various measures were taken which, however, proved more or less ineffective, but in 1915 the Local Government Board issued the Public Health (Shell-fish) Regulations, which empower any authority of the district in which the layings are situated to close

[1] See p. 19.

layings liable to sewage pollution. The procedure in the case of Liverpool was based on the routine and systematic examination of shell-fish taken at fish markets and retail shops for evidence of sewage contamination, and in the event of this being detected representations were made to the authority of the district from which they came, as well as to the wholesaler and retailer concerned, and their sale stopped.

The two methods, chemical and bacteriological, wholly distinct in their technique, supplement each other and have the same ultimate aims; broadly speaking, chemical methods are generally applicable to articles of food comprised under the term "groceries", the bacteriological to perishable articles; both are necessary in safeguarding the public from fraud, imposition and danger.

The Act required an inspector, or his agent, after purchase of a sample, to proclaim his or her identity to the vendor, offer to divide the sample into three parts, each being officially sealed, and to leave one with the vendor so that if he chose he could have an analysis made on his own behalf by another analyst. The third sample was held in reserve for subsequent independent analysis by a Home Office expert in the event of dispute. Experience proved the need for the employment of trained and practised persons for the purposes of the Act, especially in procuring samples and submitting them for analysis.

Many instances of great ingenuity in fraudulent devices have been brought to light.

A systematic analysis of a whole series of proprietary medicines showed them to contain no substance of medicinal value but they were nevertheless harmless; others, however, intended for infants and young children, contained more or less active medicinal agents, such as morphia, and were harmful; "wine" sold as a tonic without any suggestion of the alcoholic strength was dealt with. In cases such as these no question was raised as to the nature or composition of the patented medicine, and no action was taken unless actively injurious ingredients were found.

Much attention has been concentrated, both from the chemical and bacteriological points of view, on milk. Obviously the adulteration with water or the abstraction of cream, or the addition of injurious preservative, all of which would be revealed by chemical analysis, would seriously affect the value of milk as an article of diet; from the bacteriological point of view the freshness of the article and the absence of foreign bacteria, notably the typhoid bacillus or the tubercle bacillus, are supremely important.

In 1895 a Royal Commission was appointed which expressed its considered opinion that the consumption of tuberculous milk was a contributory factor to human tuberculosis.[1] The Council in 1896 engaged the services of four of the most eminent bacteriologists of the day, namely, Boyce of Liverpool, Hamilton of Aberdeen, Delépine of Manchester, and Sims Woodhead of Cambridge, to examine and report upon samples of milk taken in Liverpool in the ordinary course of delivery for human consumption. Their results showed first, that tuberculous milk was being sold, and second, that whilst 5 per cent. of the samples of milk of cows kept within the city were found to be infected, this was the case in no less than 13·4 per cent. of the samples of milk from various neighbouring counties from which about half of the city's supplies were derived. The condition of the cowsheds in the rural areas supplying milk to Liverpool was in fact analogous to that of the ill-ventilated court houses in the town—dark and dirty with vitiated atmosphere, and with the addition of accumulated filth in their vicinity. They were under no systematic supervision and were the foci of tuberculous infection.

These facts led to a close co-operation of the Liverpool cow-keepers with the Health Department, and they also led the Council to apply to Parliament in the Liverpool Act of 1900 for special powers to visit and inspect country cowsheds from which tuberculous milk was sent into Liverpool, with a view to prohibit such importation until such time as the cowsheds were put into proper order and diseased animals eliminated. Incidentally this Act of 1900 ensured the protection of the consumer from milk contaminated by filth, a necessary measure, quite apart from the question of the specific infection by the tubercle bacilli,

[1] See p. 72.

a question upon which bacteriologists were not wholly unanimous.

The Corporation of Manchester had already made application to Parliament for powers to visit and inspect country cowsheds from which tuberculous milk was supplied, and many of the great centres of population subsequently followed this course. These measures had a particularly wholesome effect upon the milk supply of the country.

Early in 1907 another Royal Commission on Tuberculosis, which had continued its inquiries since its appointment in 1901, issued its Second Interim Report. One of the conclusions is as follows:

A very considerable amount of disease and loss of life, especially among the young, must be attributed to the consumption of cows' milk containing tubercle bacilli. The milk coming from such a cow ought not to form part of human food, and indeed ought not to be used as food at all.

The possibility of such infection was controverted by Robert Koch, one of the most eminent of bacteriologists, and it was not until subsequent investigation, carried on until the Washington Congress of 1908, that Robert Koch, and others who had shared his original views, changed their opinion and agreed that an important factor in the production of tuberculosis, especially in children, is the milk of the diseased dairy cow.

Clearly, general legislation on the subject was necessary, for it was found that when the diseased milk could no longer find its way into protected areas many farmers sent it to unprotected areas, and neglected the sanitation of the cowsheds, it being frequently alleged that the farmers dare not complain to their landlords, and in any case the landlords would do nothing.

These incidents give one more illustration of the value of the initiative of the great centres of population in regard to public health legislation.

The value of the systematic examination of cows by veterinary surgeons has long been recognised; in Liverpool such provision has been available since 1898, and many cowkeepers at their own expense have caused systematic examination of their herds to be made with a view to exclude cows suffering from tubercular disease of the udder. The Liverpool Act of 1900 made obligatory the attendance of the veterinary surgeon in carrying out the Act; the importance of this procedure is evident. The Report of the Royal Commission on Tuberculosis already referred to states: "There is far less difficulty in recognising clinically that a cow is distinctly suffering from tuberculosis, in which case she may be yielding tuberculous milk", than with the bacteriological procedure.

No single article of food has received an amount of legislative and administrative attention at all comparable to that given to milk; a long succession of enactments and orders of the Local Government Board and Ministry of Health has been issued in regard to it, the first series of these, the Dairies, Cowsheds and Milkshops Orders, 1875 to 1899, have not failed to produce a lasting benefit to the community. In recent years the more efficient control of milk supplies has been secured under Acts and Regulations[1] which call for the sanitation of cowsheds, and safeguard the handling of milk from the source on the farm until delivery to the consumer. During the last few years the question of the use of preservatives in foodstuffs has been under consideration by the Government, and the recently issued Public Health (Preservatives in Food) Regulations, 1926, 1928, dealing with this subject also prevent the use in milk and other foodstuffs of preservatives or colouring matters which are deleterious to health.

Very valuable results have followed the work of the Royal Commission on Local Government (1923) whose final Report was issued in 1929, and "which has had the singular gratification of seeing many of its recommendations adopted and passed into law". The Food and Drugs Act of 1928 consolidated without amendments all the previous Acts, together with the appointment of public analysts and the legislative measures included in the many orders made under the Milk and Dairies Act.

---

[1] Milk and Dairies (Consolidation) Act, 1915; Milk and Dairies (Amendment) Act, 1922; Milk (Special Designation) Orders, 1922 and 1923; Milk and Dairies Order, 1926; and several others.

Arsenic in Beer

Towards the latter half of the year 1900 there was found to be an increase in the number of persons seeking hospital relief on account of a form of disease usually associated with alcoholic poisoning (peripheral neuritis), but in many cases the paralysis was accompanied with more or less marked pigmentation of the skin. During the same period there was also an increase, notably among women, in the ordinary cases of alcoholism, and a larger proportion than usual were attended with fatal results. The circumstance, however, was attributed to misspending of money given for the support of the families of South African Reservists. However, towards the end of November a light was suddenly thrown upon these cases by the report of Dr Reynolds of Manchester, to the effect that he had found that similar cases coming under his care in the Workhouse Hospital there were unquestionably cases of arsenical poisoning, due, as he proved, to the presence of arsenic in beer. This discovery by Dr Reynolds at once aroused the suspicion of the possibility of arsenic being present in beer in Liverpool, although the reports of the City Analyst had not suggested this contamination, samples submitted for analysis during October having been certified to be genuine; in view however of the quantities of beer consumed in some districts of the city, it was obvious that if arsenic were present, nothing but the promptest measures could avert a calamity.

A large number of samples of beer were at once purchased in different parts of the city and submitted to immediate qualitative analysis, and the results showed that 20 per cent. of certain brews were contaminated with arsenic; in each case the whole of the beer upon the premises concerned, and which might by any possibility be suspected of contamination, was ordered to be forthwith run into the sewers, or the barrels were sealed up with the official seal in use in taking samples under the Sale of Food and Drugs Act, and their contents emptied into the sewers as soon as practicable. With a single exception the brewers showed anxiety that any beer suspected of arsenical contamination should be withdrawn from the market, and themselves employed analysts of repute to assist in the matter owing to the rush of work thrown on the City Analyst and his staff in endeavouring to locate the source of the mischief. The single exception alluded to was a Manchester firm and otherwise a reputable one, but means were promptly found to bring that firm to its senses, and the destruction of the beer completed.

At the time the procedure gave rise to some criticism on the grounds that proceedings were not taken under the Sale of Food and Drugs Act, as would be the case in the vendor of any other article known or suspected to be contaminated with arsenic. The situation, however, called for instant action, and delay consequent upon procedure under the Sale of Food and Drugs Act, which involved quantitative analysis and the subsequent legal procedure, would have had very serious consequences upon the health of the beer drinker. The legal procedure which did follow was on civil grounds and was not instituted by the Public Health Department.

The main source of arsenic was found to be glucose, manufactured from an impure sulphuric acid containing arsenic, supplied by a Leeds firm.

The actual number of authenticated cases of arsenical poisoning in Liverpool at no time reached as high a figure as in Manchester, but the number of definite cases was 102, and the number of known fatal cases 3. In all likelihood, however, the actual numbers were somewhat in excess of these figures.

Supervision of Meat

The earliest efforts to deal with food supplies were indirect and dealt in the main with the nuisance arising from slaughtering of animals, and the conveyance through the streets of animals smothered or damaged during the voyage from Ireland. In 1828 a person was appointed termed a leavelooker ("leave to look") to take note of the character of the meat, and later a depot was established to which injured and smothered cattle were removed.

The Act of 1842—"an Act for the improvement, good government and police regulation of the Borough of Liverpool" —contained clauses dealing with the handling of meat, the regulating and registration of existing slaughter-houses, the licensing of new ones, the appointment of inspectors of slaughter-houses and meat, and the cleanly conveyance of meat through the streets.

In the case of any inspector of slaughter-houses finding any cattle, or the carcasses or part of the carcass of any cattle smothered or injured in transport, "it shall be lawful for the inspector to seize and take, and carry away, any unsound or unwholesome meat, or direct the same to be seized, taken and carried away, by any servant or assistant, for the purpose of being further examined by competent persons according to the usual course and practice heretofore adopted in the borough". This was a jury of three members of the trade. Each member received a gratuity of 1s. 6d. and signed a certificate. The object was to protect the inspector from any charge of irregularity to which, however, the system rather lent itself. This practice was not wholly discontinued until about the year 1900, it then, however, applied only to meat voluntarily given up and had an altogether different significance, namely, to imply that the trade agreed in the view of the inspector and no magisterial action was necessary.

Places of deposit for smothered cattle were fixed, and masters of vessels were required to give information regarding smothered cattle, whilst Justices were empowered to order carcasses to be burned or destroyed to prevent them being used for food, and the inspectors were empowered to inspect meat hawked about for sale. These well-considered requirements were pushed into the background by other and more urgent calls, notably epidemic disease, which absorbed almost the whole attention of the Council.[1]

In 1851 the need for minimising the number of slaughtering places became manifest, and the principles laid down by Mr Newlands that abattoirs should be placed in the open country, and that the driving of animals and oxen through the crowded thoroughfares interrupting traffic and endangering the public should be avoided, were approved by the Council but no action was taken.

After many years of contention and discussion, and as a consequence of the ever-growing evil, the trade opposition was

[1] See Chapter II.

ultimately overcome, and finally in 1927 the City Council decided to proceed with the much-needed abattoir in an appropriate situation suitably adjacent to railway sidings and contiguous to the Stanley Cattle Market: the building is now in full progress. The gain to the city from this step will be immense.

When the Public Health Act of 1875 was enacted certain clauses were incorporated dealing with the inspection of meat and meat foods and they became the main clauses under which the supervision of food has been carried out.

With regard to the importation of cattle, mainly from Ireland, transport was rough and the animals ill-cared for. The late Mr Alfred Booth was active in securing the provision of regulations designed to protect the animals, cattle, pigs and sheep, from injury and suffering during the voyage. Close supervision was exercised by the Liverpool Port Sanitary Authority.

The enormous importation of chilled and frozen meat was effectively controlled by regulations issued in the year 1908, one set of which, designated the Unsound Food Regulations, dealt with unsound food of all classes including meat.

These regulations, which were strengthened from time to time in order to meet evasions, have had the effect of reducing the amount of diseased and unsound food coming into the port of Liverpool in a remarkable manner.

In the large ports of this country, and particularly Liverpool, owing to stress of weather or accidents of the voyage it is obvious that consignments of meat, grain, and fruit, must from time to time arrive in an unsound or unsaleable condition. These are all dealt with by a fully trained staff capable of dealing with every condition which may arise.

The damaged food is frequently allowed to go for industrial purposes or for the manufacture of poultry feeding stuffs or size making, or in the manufacture of agricultural fertilisers; if incapable of being used in these ways it is destroyed.

The whole system has been carefully organised and has become very efficient.

Chapter XII

GENERAL EFFECTS OF PUBLIC
HEALTH LEGISLATION

PUBLIC health legislation received a great stimulus from
Edwin Chadwick, Southwood Smith, Duncan, and many
others, who in various ways emphasised the need for
powers to deal with the disease, misery and crime associated
with the unwholesome conditions of life in the great centres of
population. Those needs were nowhere more evident than in
Liverpool, and hence it is that the applications to Parliament
made by the Town Council in order to meet the many needs
are unique in frequency and variety. The usefulness of many
of the clauses so obtained became so plain as to justify their
adoption subsequently by other cities, and indeed to serve as a
basis for many of the provisions of the Public Health Act passed
many years later.

The necessity for some alteration had been strongly urged
upon Liverpool, and from many quarters she was urged to
examine into her own condition, and begin in earnest to set
it right. Mr McGowan observes that:

The principle of the Liverpool Act of 1847 was purely that of
Local Government. It entrusted enormous powers to the adminis-
trators, at the same time appointing for the office the Town Council,
comprising gentlemen of high character and intelligence—a Government sufficiently permanent to induce the members to study the
subject, popular enough to ensure a spirit of moderation, and familiar
with local exigencies. The scope of the Act was so to deal with private
rights as to make them subordinate to the public welfare.

Such is the force of good example, for so imperative had become the
necessity for similar action in other towns that the Liverpool Act
opened a new era in legislation. Two months afterwards the Baths
and Wash-houses Act was passed, as also the Nuisances Removal and
Diseases Prevention Act. In the year following the Towns Improvement Clauses Act became law, embodying most of the Liverpool
provisions. These were followed in 1848 by the Public Health Act,
the Nuisances Removal Amendment Act, and subsequently, from
time to time, by various other measures relating to the subject.

The difficulty of the problems which it was desired to solve was more fully revealed when the Corporation was clothed with authority to deal with them; supplementary legislation became necessary and important additions were from time to time made to their powers. These, *inter alia*, empowered the closure of cellars situated in courts, better control of furnaces with a view to abating the smoke nuisance, whilst provision of baths and wash-houses was facilitated.

The full effect could not be felt at once since the operations contemplated extended over several years. The displacement of the cellar population was necessarily slow, as any attempt at haste would have resulted in overcrowding other unhealthy dwellings of the court house type. The provision of baths and wash-houses was also a gradual operation, but their popularity encouraged their development.

Sewer construction proceeded apace, no less than 80 miles of sewers being constructed in the subsequent eleven years. Many sewage pits were drained or filled up, water hydrants multiplied so as to afford greater facilities for washing courts, passages and streets, and habitable cellars were registered and put under control. Some control was also exercised over the interments of the dead, and burials within Church buildings abolished or regulated. "Added to other improvements there was the great blessing of an immensely increased water supply...and as a result of this an increase of baths in private houses of moderate rental, and the gradual abandoning of cesspools." The Local Government Act of 1858 conferred greatly increased powers on the Council, especially in regard to the width and direction of streets, and the space to be allotted in and about dwelling-houses; unfortunately the advantages of these powers were not fully realised, and they were used only to a limited extent.

Then, as now, there was always an unwillingness to embark upon costly projects, or indeed upon any project unless immediate benefit could be shown, and the projects, the advantageous results of which were not immediately obvious, but which had to be waited for, were not favoured. In regard to the question of sewering, "the advantage of drainage and sewerage within the Borough has to some extent been neutralised by the existence of tracts of undrained land surrounding it. The increase of houses on this area has led to polluted water courses, which at length became uncovered sewers". The application of the General Health Act was impossible, since there was no continuous chain of townships, but there were gaps of open country between some of the then out-townships and the town of Liverpool and their inhabitants were not uniformly distributed in those outer districts, but were for the most part huddled together in the narrow streets and courts of the original village; and there was no possibility of the combination requisite to establish the continuous system of sewerage, for which a combined and controlling power was necessary. The only hope then felt was in an extension of the borough for sanitary purposes, an incorporation which had to be waited for.

In 1858 further powers were sought to deal in a more comprehensive way with the slum areas. It would appear that the failure of the Public Health Act of 1848 lay in its excessive centralisation. "The London Board were virtually the managers; their agents sometimes had an interest in the works. The local board became mere collectors of taxes, and servants obeying orders", and needless interference by those unfamiliar with the circumstances, "particularly if the interference be in the wrong direction, as not infrequently happens", led to resentment and conflict. The passing of a new Local Government Act appears to have remedied the difficulty, since it contained certain adoptive clauses which enabled the Local Authority "to apply any portion of the Act to its district", thus enabling it, without expense, to exercise powers which would otherwise have required a special Act, and in many cases would have excited fierce opposition.

Contemporaneous writers refer to the improving moral as well as physical effects which resulted from the substantial sanitary progress made, but they also mention the handicap of the circumstances attendant upon a seaport, such as:

Its being a depôt for emigrants and immigrants, containing more than the average of very wretched people; cargoes of lunatics deported from America without anyone in charge of them, casualties happening amongst shipping, and the like; miserable people attracted to the town in the hope of finding employment, intruding themselves upon an already overcrowded labour-population, and thus producing suffering and injury to health, together with an enormous amount of pauperism.[1]

It will interest persons whose occupation lies in Dale Street to know that in 1855 that street is described as "the vilest part of the Parish", a condition which is associated with the then pleasing circumstance "that Typhus, which was *formerly* the opprobrium of Liverpool, caused *only* 342 deaths".

The Liverpool Sanitary Amendment Act of 1854 made provision for improving the drainage of the outer areas of the growing town; but so far as the owners of land and builders were concerned, its application was optional, and it took some time before its advantages were realised. With regard to "made soils" the Act checked the further construction of dwellings on the refuse material from gas and general works deposited in previous years.

Instances were frequent of quarries being filled with loose earth and rubbish, and the floors of houses erected on this insecure foundation without any timber, proper footings, or any contrivance to render them stable, with all the attendant evils and expense.

The replacement of boulder streets with sets and granite curbs was finding favour, experimental methods were being tried in regard to the durability of the flagging used in the foot-walks, and places of refuge were provided at suitable crossings in order to obviate the danger arising from the street passengers crossing the streets at every point, a provision which unhappily has not been continued, notwithstanding the ever increasing need for it. The advice given by the City Engineer as to the propriety of making provision for public waiting rooms did not find acceptance.

Mr Newlands referring twelve years later to the 1846 Act says, "in certain districts, apparently near to hospitals in order to lessen the noise, sets and wooden blocks were tried in alternative courses, an arrangement, however, which by the wearing of the wood appears to have added to rather than diminished it".

[1] Reports, 1855.

Difficulties in regard to public conveniences arrested attention and a proposal to construct waiting rooms in Wapping received the approval of the Corporation, but when the plans were prepared it was found that the land was required for other purposes. A similar fate followed proposals in regard to Clayton Square, and elsewhere. "In truth there appears very little prospect in the present state of feeling on the subject, of this experiment being tried."

With regard to scavenging, anxiety of the Committee in 1853 and 1854 to have the town in the state of the greatest possible cleanliness when a visitation of the scourge of Cholera was dreaded, caused an increase in the cost of scavenging; but the active exertions anticipatory of this in improving the paving in the worst localities, had the effect of rendering the increase much the same as it otherwise would have been.

The total cost of scavenging and cleansing in the year 1853 was £9758. 1s. 9d., in 1856 it was £12,127.[1]

By 1851, 20,000 inmates had been ejected from the deeper cellar dwellings, which were mostly damp and filthy. Then, as in later years, great opposition arose to the closure of insanitary dwellings, one reason being the reluctance of the inmates to leave their miserable abodes, a reluctance chiefly founded on the convenience offered by the separate entrance to the cellars, and the facilities for selling cakes, fruit, vegetables, chips, etcetera. "So strong is this feeling that were it not for the constant and systematic inspection of the officers employed for this special purpose under the Inspector of Nuisances, the cellars would be re-occupied nearly as fast as they are cleared." In 18,000 cases the occupants were summoned before the magistrate, and in 2386 cases, cellars which had been re-occupied after having been cleared, were cleared a second time. To bring the cellar within the provision of the Act proof had to be given of its occupation by night, and in order to withhold this proof the parties were in the habit of concealing in the day-time the straw or shavings which they used as bedding.[2]

The 1860 Report was the last written by Dr Duncan, to whose magnificent work the city owes so much. In that final report he

---

answers the hostile criticisms of expenditure on health matters by pointing out that "expenditure on sanitation had borne abundant fruit, and pointed not without satisfaction to the fact that Typhus Fever had caused *only* 359 deaths against the previous ten years average of 540".

The Registrar General's return shows that the actual total number of deaths was as great as it is to-day with a population more than twice as large; the Report concludes:

looking at these results, and remembering that before the passing of the Liverpool Sanitary Act the annual mortality of Liverpool was notoriously and invariably higher than that of any other town in the kingdom, the authorities and rate-payers may congratulate themselves that the expenditure for sanitary purposes since 1847—large as it has been—has borne abundant fruit, and that the results have been made commensurate with the sacrifices which have been made. It may be hoped that the disparaging remarks which have been made from time to time, as to the results of sanitary operations in Liverpool, may henceforward cease, and that even the most unreasonable may be satisfied that the proceedings of the Health Committee have been productive of Benefit.

Subsequent applications to Parliament to amend and strengthen existing Acts have been frequent, almost annual, and in many instances they preceded general legislation relating to similar objects. The powers sought were almost invariably granted by Parliament and in some of the rare instances in which the applications were refused they were granted subsequently. The Liverpool Sanitary Amendment Act of 1864, as has already been pointed out, facilitated operations designed to deal with insanitary dwellings, the Liverpool Sanitary Act of 1866 included clauses dealing with sub-letting, the Public Health Act of 1866, amongst other things, authorised the provision of hospitals, a subject dealt with elsewhere, and the Liverpool Improvement Act of 1867 controlled the keeping of cows and also the keeping of pigs.

It is not necessary to follow in detail the various provisions relating to public health which were inserted in the numerous applications made to Parliament, references to them will be found in the sections to which they refer; the whole of these provisions are now consolidated in the Liverpool Act of 1921.

General legislation has still further facilitated the task of all Sanitary Authorities, and so far as Liverpool is concerned, the city has fully availed itself of them.

The Local Government Act of 1929 affords many opportunities to the Council for advancing public health administration since it supplements the well-tried methods of *prevention* of disease by adding to the facilities for *treatment*; transferring, in fact, the whole of the Poor Law Hospital system from the Boards of Guardians to the Council; the power now given to the Council to provide hospital accommodation to meet ordinary necessities corresponds with the power to provide accommodation for infectious sickness. A very wide field is opened since hospital accommodation is needed for classes other than those formerly under Poor Law relief. Hitherto the Poor Law Authorities, through workhouses and Poor Law institutions, were required to provide for the poor alone, although no doubt many who did not come under the category of "paupers" benefited very largely by the Poor Law administration, and one of the results of the transfer will be to extend this class.

The Act provides facilities for infusing into the conduct of the hospitals much of the tone, method of staffing, and so forth, which have proved so valuable in voluntary general or special hospitals. The question of admission of the patient will depend upon the medical certificate, the question of pauperism being eliminated.

Recovery of expenses is an important consideration, but any method adopted in a hospital controlled by a Council which would place obstacles in the way of a sick person who is in need of hospital treatment from receiving it will be avoided. A lesson, in fact, in this direction may be learnt from the long experiences of infectious diseases hospitals; at one time there was a feeling in favour of making a charge for admission inasmuch as the Public Health Act authorised such charge, but it was found to be a futile and objectionable procedure, and the proposals were dropped; the point may possibly be met by a method of insurance. The help and co-operation of the medical profession may be safely relied upon in any difficulties which may arise.

Index

Principal references in heavier type

Index

Printed in the United States
By Bookmasters